Praise for
The Language of Breath

"As a society, we have been driven to strive and achieve, making the desire to accumulate our main priority and losing ourselves in the process. With our limited time and breath, we push our health to the limit and sacrifice ourselves to the pursuit of an idealized happiness. In *The Language of Breath*, Jesse Coomer brings the reader's awareness back to the breath and body and out of our heads. When we get out of our heads and focus on the world around us, we can connect more with the beauty and intelligence of life. The result is a reduction in stress, greater happiness, and learning to live life according to one's true self. What a gift!"

—PATRICK MCKEOWN, author *The Oxygen Advantage*

"If you have any interest in breathwork, this is an essential book for your library."

—CHUCK MCGEE III, breathwork instructor and ACT practitioner

"An inveterate breathworker and biohacker, Coomer provides valuable insights on how breathing changes the way we interact with the world. We are walking miracles and it's our privilege to explore ourselves."

—SCOTT CARNEY, *New York Times* best-selling author of *What Doesn't Kill Us*

"Jesse Coomer is one of the world's foremost breathing experts, and he has managed in this book to gather some of the best-of-the-best techniques that you must know if you want to become a true breathwork ninja. I highly recommend you add this book to your physiology library to learn how to use your breath to create a powerful connection within yourself so that you can take powerful actions in the world around you!"

—BEN GREENFIELD, human performance consultant at BenGreenfieldLife.com

"Jesse has taken a complex and intricate subject and turned it into a simple yet insightful philosophy that has systematically helped me understand the key to the mind-body connection. The Listening Exercises teaches you to filter through the noise of the egoic mind and how to pay attention and listen to the language of the breath and uncover the answers you desire."

—MARTIN MCPHILIMEY, BSc (Hons), MSc, Mres, consultant and respiratory and sleep scientist at Performance Through Health

"In *The Language of Breath,* Jesse Coomer provides a clear path for how to implement all forms of breathwork in the current breathwork spectrum [and] a narrative journey that educates as much as it inspires. In his detailed history of not only breathwork, but also the treatment of disease, Coomer motivates and provides efficacy of practice in each chapter . . . with several examples of applications for everyday individuals who would like to use breathwork to better their lives. A gifted educator who expresses his passion for breathwork and helping others, Coomer offers a book that is as enjoyable to read as it is educational."

—AJ FISHER, founder of Hypoxix.fitness | @ajcorectology

"Right from the start, Coomer's unique take on our relationship to breathing expresses something deeply profound that is not easily put into words. This book not only gives us a new way to learn how to listen to the body, it also teaches us ways to *respond* to it kindly. The book overflows with powerful, *original* practices—a rare thing!"

—TOM GRANGER, author of *Draw Breath*

"There is no mistake that you have found Jesse Coomer's book—his teachings are definitely a blessing we are all receiving. *The Language of Breath* is filled with tools for those who want to take control of their nervous system (and life) and become more aware of their thoughts—which control everything around us. Coomer is the real deal, and his willingness to be of service is what the world needs. [In this book] you might find a better way to live life with joy, cease resistance to reality, and learn how to control the outcomes."

—BEATRIZ BOAS, founder of Theta Breathwork™

"The world doesn't need more breathing techniques; it needs more inclusive ways for you to find what works for you! Jesse brings his profound experience in teaching both language and breath together in a wonderful road map for self-exploration. With this great guidebook, you can stop looking for more information, techniques, or methods on how to breathe and start speaking the language of your own body."

—KASPER VAN DER MEULEN, "The Breathwork Biohacker," www.BreathworkMasterclass.com

THE
LANGUAGE
OF BREATH

THE LANGUAGE OF BREATH

Discover Better
Emotional and Physical
Health through Breathing
and Self-Awareness

JESSE COOMER

FOREWORD BY BRIAN MACKENZIE
AFTERWORD BY RICHARD BOSTOCK

North Atlantic Books
Huichin, unceded Ohlone land
Berkeley, California

Published by
North Atlantic Books
Huichin, unceded Ohlone land
Berkeley, California

Cover design by Carlos Esparza
Book design by Happenstance Type-O-Rama

Printed in the United States of America

The Language of Breath: Discover Better Emotional and Physical Health through Breathing and Self-Awareness is sponsored and published by North Atlantic Books, an educational non-profit based in the unceded Ohlone land Huichin (Berkeley, CA) that collaborates with partners to develop cross-cultural perspectives; nurture holistic views of art, science, the humanities, and healing; and seed personal and global transformation by publishing work on the relationship of body, spirit, and nature.

North Atlantic Books' publications are distributed to the US trade and internationally by Penguin Random House Publisher Services. For further information, visit our website at www.northatlanticbooks.com.

Library of Congress Cataloging-in-Publication Data

Names: Coomer, Jesse, 1980– author.
Title: The language of breath : discover better emotional and physical
   health through breathing and self-awareness / by Jesse Coomer.
Description: Berkeley, California : North Atlantic Books, [2023] | Includes
   bibliographical references and index.
Identifiers: LCCN 2023010441 (print) |, LCCN 2023010442 (ebook) | ISBN
   9781623179366 (trade paperback) | ISBN 9781623179373 (ebook) | ISBN
   9781623179373 (ebook)
Subjects: LCSH: Breathing exercises—Therapeutic use. | Mind and body. |
   Mindfulness (Psychology) | Self-help techniques.
Classification: LCC RM733 .C66 2023 (print) | LCC RM733 (ebook) | DDC
   613/.192—dc23/eng/20230605
LC record available at https://lccn.loc.gov/2023010441
LC ebook record available at https://lccn.loc.gov/2023010442

1 2 3 4 5 6 7 8 9 KPC 28 27 26 25 24 23

CONTENTS

FOREWORD

BRIAN MACKENZIE

Breathing is the most fundamental aspect of nature and, therefore, human nature. After all, we are nature. I have found nothing else to be more precise or closer to the truth. When I do, I will make sure to share that. I found out all this through human performance.

My background in human performance came from sport and a deep connection to water, namely the ocean. I began teaching and coaching professionally in early 2000, getting a deeper understanding of human movement through running mechanics, endurance performance, altitude training, adaptive physical education, and working as a physical therapy assistant. Around 2004 I began implementing Ashtanga yoga into my weekly training routine to offset the rigors of my training ideas around endurance. I was introduced to breath control and its application to movement, but I would largely ignore this fundamental aspect of movement with breathing for some time. By 2007, I had studied and had a pretty good grasp on strength and conditioning—something I had successfully implemented into endurance work. Most of my career revolved around applying physical stressors and movement principles.

One would think that I missed the opportunity to realize how breathing could have played a role in everything, but that would be incorrect, as I have come to understand. It was always there, but back then, I was in no way capable of understanding what I do now. Nonetheless, my pivot to breathing came via a resistance breathing device.

I laughed at the claim that it could change altitude or pressure enough to do anything for low oxygen adaptations, but I put it on anyway. In doing so, I learned that the pressure this mask provided changed much more than

I understood (maybe not oxygen levels). This moment—and I remember it vividly—changed everything in my career and my life, and I knew it at that moment.

I began playing with and testing many ideas quickly: some bizarre, some rational; others took time. However, the more I experimented, the more I learned, and the more I learned, the more books I continued to read on physiology and biology surrounding the respiratory system, metabolism, and ultimately the nervous system.

I met Jesse Coomer when I was teaching at a breath seminar in Los Angeles. Looking back, the seminar was too narrowly focused on just one way of thinking about breath. I'm not going to lie. It felt a little culty. What is most interesting about our meeting is that, since then, we have both explored this breathing thing far more profoundly than that weekend could have ever provided. However, were it not for that weekend, neither of us would be where we are, and I certainly would not be here to tell you about the importance of this book.

If I had not done the work that breathing led me to, I'd probably be jealous. This is practically the book I envisioned myself writing on breathing and its impact on us. So, this is all to say, Jesse Coomer has done his homework, and even more apparent is that he has done *the* work. And I want to be clear that I am delighted he has done it.

Today what exists in the ecosystem of this space surrounding breath and meditation could be compared to the nutrition space. Think of it like this:

- Most people are teaching and participating in fast food–like remedies to meet caloric needs and quick fixes. This is much like what you will find in the click-bait articles online about breathwork. "Just one simple trick to eliminate stress!"

- Some are aware they will probably need to eat real food but cling to ideologies like paleo, vegan, vegetarian, or low-carb, carving out space to do a particular method. In the breathwork space, this is much like those who espouse a single school of breathwork or who have a cult-like devotion to one specific technique.

- Then there begins to be a separation for a select few where the science gets meaningful but remains a little ideological, doing only what research states, never exploring the edges or what works for individuals. We see this rigidness in breath all the time as well.

- On the far end of nutrition and any work involving biology is biochemistry and the art of interpreting the individual and what foods may work, may not work, could be causing problems, or not. The exciting thing about biochemistry is that breath influences and responds to it 24 hours per day, 7 days per week, 365 days per year. This is where academia, science, understanding, and practice begin to converge, and teaching and learning become an art form.

What lies ahead in this manual is a path to understanding how to navigate how you operate and how to use the most potent tool and lever we have for understanding some of our most profound truths. As you are about to read, breathing is the most fundamental part of our being, as it is intimately tied to cellular respiration and the most critical aspect of all life: energy. If we stop producing energy effectively—which is quite a rabbit hole—we begin to experience aging and disease at accelerated rates. The oversimplified version of this is that cellular respiration is far more than just moving energy, as it produces and manages proteins and nucleotides responsible for the very building blocks of life, of our lives. When the flux of energy peters out, we die. We must transfer energy effectively as everything in this universe requires it, and we are as much a part of that process as everything else. We are simply subject to the human version of that.

Our minds are restless, we have isolated ourselves, and we are not doing well. We are ill. *The Language of Breath* offers guidance for meeting yourself for the first time. This is an opportunity to see how the pipes are getting clogged and how to understand your health. Jesse has masterfully outlined this process along with our nervous system and the relationship to carbon dioxide, oxygen's greatest asset. He understands that stress is killing us and that our physiology is communicating to us to take action. I was someone who had no idea what he was getting into so many years ago with this breathing thing, but

I knew it would lead me to something revolutionary. It did—the very things that *The Language of Breath* details.

I do not hope you find what I have found here. Nor do I hope you find what Jesse has. Instead, I would love for you to find yourself and how powerful you are with this book as your guide.

INTRODUCTION

THE MODERN HUMAN CONDITION

A common joke in offices and libraries around the United States is, "It is okay to talk to yourself, just as long as you don't answer back." It is normally said after someone apologizes for talking to themselves out loud, which can be a bit confusing in an office full of people. This joke is usually made by the same person who says things like "You won't get far without those" when someone forgets their keys, or "Is it hot enough for ya?" in the summer.

The reality is that we are all engaged in one form of self-talk or another, whether we are speaking out loud or not. This book is dedicated to deciphering a form of self-talk that most of us don't realize we are doing, a constant stream of communication that affects everything from our mood to our blood pressure to our ability to laugh politely when someone makes a worn-out joke at the office. In the twenty-first century, there has never been a greater need to be aware of this inner communication, a quality of being human that we are only just now becoming aware of.

The human condition is a term used to refer to all the qualities, experiences, events, and feelings that permeate the entire human species, from the earliest time in our history to the present. The feeling of loneliness, birth, death, and longing for love have been expressed in poetry, painting, songs, and theater for as long as these media have existed, sharing the common human experience across the ages. However, modern humans are slowly becoming aware of a new shared condition, one that is a distinct hallmark of our place on the technological timeline.

For decades, we have become more painfully aware of a disconnection between ourselves and the modern artificial world that we are now seemingly encased within. In the time since the Industrial Revolution, it became clear that humans living in modernized environments were suffering from previously unaccounted-for ailments. We put humans in small, poorly ventilated spaces, left them to sit and do repetitive tasks, and treated them like the machines they were paid to operate. In the twentieth century, major advancements in food preservation, air-conditioning, communication, and transportation ushered in an era where our species began to live in an environment and under daily conditions that were even more alien to our biology. While advancements in technology offered amenities that were more comfortable and much safer, with regard to many of the dangers of our past, decade after decade we have seen more and more of the unforeseen negative impacts of living in the modern world.

Where starvation was once a very real threat to the average human's lifespan, modern humans face the ills of abundance, with approximately one in ten Americans suffering from type 2 diabetes[1] and another one in three Americans prediabetic.[2] Where we once worked ourselves to early deaths hunting, gathering, and farming, the average American spends 55 percent of waking hours completely sedentary.[3] We don't seem to be able to sleep like we used to,[4] we spend billions of dollars each year because we can't seem to digest our food like we once did,[5] and according to wide population-based studies, 33 percent of the population will suffer from an anxiety disorder in their lifetime—a sobering statistic, especially considering the fact that anxiety disorders are often not recognized or reported.[6]

While it is clear that modern life offers many incredible benefits that we would not want to give up there seems to be a disconnection between the biological creatures we are and the modern environment we live in, a phenomenon that seems to have finally caught up with our advances in medicine, leading to recent drops in life expectancy for those who are being born now over previous generations.[7]

The modern human condition is one of a strange disconnection. However, because we assume that the way things are today is "normal," we have a difficult time understanding what is happening to us. We fear what we don't understand, especially when it is ourselves. The reality is that we modern humans unknowingly suffer from a misunderstanding about what we are and how we interact with our environments. And what we do not know is causing us harm.

My Story, Our Story

The modern human condition described above was the story of my life for my first thirty years. Like most modern humans, I had no foundational understanding of my own species. I was born into a modern environment, asked to sit at a school desk for twelve years, and then sent to more desks in more artificial environments, without any substantial advice on how my nervous system works or accurate explanations of what emotions are or how to manage them. In fact, much of the discussion about what makes us human was often with regard for how much we are like machines. This is a destructive paradigm that we will discuss in the first chapter of this book.

All this misunderstanding about myself led me to not trust myself. I couldn't trust how I felt; I didn't even know why I felt the way I felt. I only knew that I was often more nervous than confident, more likely to overthink than to be in a state of flow, and more likely to choke in moments of stress than to step into opportunities with confidence. In my late teens and early twenties, like so many people, I decided that the best way to deal with my anxiety and lack of confidence was simply not to try. At least then I wouldn't have to choke and fail. Of course, this only led me to further self-disconnection, which led me to trying to control the way I felt with drugs and alcohol. It wasn't until the end of my twenties, when I began to reconnect with myself, that I began a journey to discover what I wish I had been told when I was a child.

Somehow, I made it through graduate school and became a professor of English. Today, I am a recovering college professor of over a decade. I have seen firsthand the effects of the modern world on the mental health of our youth. When I began teaching, smart phones were not seen in the classroom, and in my last years of teaching, they were ubiquitous, along with more complaints about stress, sleepless nights, and self-destructive behavior. Of course, I was just as stressed out as my students, and so was everyone else. Even in

2015, The *Journal of the American Medical Association* cited that 60 to 80 percent of primary care visits had a stress-related component and that 44 percent of Americans reported experiencing more stress in the past five years.[8] In my attempts to deal with my own struggles with stress and anxiety, I eventually stumbled on breathwork. My life has never been the same.

When I discovered breathwork, I couldn't believe it was actually "a thing." To be honest, I still wake up every morning, blown away that this incredible method of self-communication is real! For the longest time I thought it was some kind of magic. Of course, it is often marketed as *actual* magic, much to my disappointment. I would say it is magic in the same sense that a beautiful sunrise is magic. Or perhaps it is magic in the way that I find my wife to be magic. But these things are not imaginary things like fairies and pixie dust. They are very real, just like the way breathing works is very real.

The practice of breathwork goes back thousands of years, but the scientific connection between breathing and mental and physical health can be traced back to the American Civil War when Dr. Da Costa unwittingly documented the first breathing disorder. He observed three hundred soldiers who suffered from what would, in the early 1900s, be dubbed hyperventilation syndrome, a breathing disorder that is common today. The twentieth century saw a steady rise in research into how breathing influences the autonomic nervous system (ANS). The ANS regulates our heart rate, our digestive system, our reproductive organs, blood sugar, and a whole host of systems within us over which we do not have conscious control. When these organs are regulated in a manner that is disconnected from how we consciously would like to use them, we suffer many of the ills of what I have dubbed "the modern human condition." As of today, there are vast numbers of studies confirming the effect that breathing (for better or worse) has on our overall health, how it allows us to consciously influence our autonomic nervous system,[9] and how it can be used to relieve emotional anxiety.[10] This scientific understanding of how breathing works has offered us an opportunity to improve our lives with every breath we take.

Today, breathwork as a practice is blooming, and there are many voices in the emerging world of breathwork. Many of these voices are excellent, but many oversimplify how breathing works or focus only on one technique or style of breathing to the exclusion of the rest. Sadly, as was the case with the fitness industry in the early days, there are also lots of claims made today about breathwork that are exaggerations and outright lies. Just like there is no pill that will make you attractive, there is no breathwork technique that will make it so that you are never sick again, never feel sad, or never have a bad day.

Breathwork will not change your life for you, but when you learn how it works, you can enjoy a state where you can creatively and confidently take better actions. It is your actions that will lead you to a better life. This is the amazing value that a holistic approach to breathwork can offer. In fact, much of the self-doubt that I experienced as a youth, which led me to avoid trying just to avoid failure, could have been ameliorated if I had just known how to interpret the way I was feeling and respond with my breathing.

Since 2016 I have been a professional breathworker, and I have trained clients from all around the world who are dealing with a long list of modern issues that all stem from the same disconnections that I see in nearly all modern people. In that time, I have trained first responders, CEOs, athletes, recovering addicts, and people from every walk of life who deserve to understand themselves in a way that will allow them to reconnect to themselves and take actions with more thoughtfulness, confidence, and focus. This same training is in the pages of this book, and it is my hope that you will also become a more connected individual as a result of reading it.

What to Expect from the Language of Breath

The Language of Breath Philosophy outlined in this book is based on the ancient practices of controlled breathing that have been documented and passed down for thousands of years, the scientific research that has been done for over one hundred years, and my years of experience that I have accumulated helping people improve their lives and form a better relationship within themselves. While the concept of communication within us might sound a bit esoteric, the reality is that it is all based on your innate biological desire to survive and thrive within the world and within your culture. You deserve to understand how this works, and I will do my best to explain it as I have come to understand it from time spent in research and after numerous occasions interacting with intellectuals and academics in the field of psychology and neuroscience. We know that there is an incredible amount of information that is always being sent and received within us. The skills you will learn in this book will allow you to take an active part in this process.

In the first three chapters, I will challenge you to see yourself differently than you might see yourself now. Much of the disconnection we experience in the modern age is built on misconceptions that have been handed down over generations. These misconceptions have been with us for so long that we simply don't think about them. They are embedded in the very language that we use to describe ourselves. For many adopters of breathwork, their experience is hampered by a fundamental misunderstanding about themselves, and therefore they always see breathwork through the wrong lens. The entire book is dedicated to correcting this misunderstanding, so don't worry if you have trouble letting go of the old paradigm early on.

We will begin your training by learning to become aware of the unconscious-self's subtle messages. In chapters 4 and 5, you will learn how to become aware of your unconscious-self and how to decipher its subtle language. In chapter 6, you will learn how to send your first message. In chapter 7, you'll learn how functional breathing adds proper tone and inflection to the communications you send in every breath. In chapter 8, we start to combine what we have learned into the foundational exercise, the Awareness Exercise. In chapter 9, we develop a breathing vocabulary, using a variety of techniques. Chapter 10 answers the question, should I breathe through my nose or my mouth? Chapters 11 and 12 cover ways that you can strengthen your inner relationship even further by raising your CO_2 tolerance or using superventilation, taking your unconscious-self to the gym, or interrupting it when it won't stop talking. Chapter 13 explains the biological function of emotions and offers a powerful exercise to connect with the unconscious-self to hear what it has to say, offering a powerful way to make connections that we might never have known existed.

The last chapter is dedicated to helping you use everything you learn in this book to form a daily practice and to make positive changes to your life. Whether it is to improve athletic performance, to become more comfortable in social situations, to increase creativity, or simply to deal with times when you cannot take action, I've got some starter plans for you there. In nearly every chapter there is an exercise or practical advice on how to master each lesson as we get closer to creating the positive relationship within you that you deserve to have.

Starting with chapter 3, you will find Language Labs at the end of each chapter with guidance on how to implement what you have learned. These skills take some time to acquire, so don't get in a rush. The foundational skills you will learn in the early chapters will pay dividends as you progress, and everything you learn will serve as a foundation that you will build on in subsequent chapters. While you can read the book straight through, you might consider taking a day or two between these chapters to practice the skills in each so that you are ready to build on them in the next chapter. It is up to you, but if you chose to practice the skills for a couple of days to a week between chapters after chapter 4, you will likely gain a more profound understanding of the material.

Having a healthy relationship with yourself and your environment is your birthright. This book is dedicated to helping you learn the method of self-connection that has served my clients and my own practice for years, helping one human at a time become more connected and more capable of taking positive actions. Breathwork will not take those actions for you, but when you learn to use your breathing as a language, you will learn to communicate with yourself in a way that will help you to think more clearly and act with greater confidence. May every breath you take bring you a greater connection.

Misconceptions Lead to Disconnections

A book published in the eleventh century called *The Almanac of Health* tells the story of an elderly man who went to his doctor one winter day complaining of achy joints and a general feeling of cold. After examining his patient, the doctor prescribed a rooster. Since it is a hot and dry bird, the doctor considered it the ideal remedy for an old man in such a condition. This is an example of the application of one of the most enduring misconceptions in the history of medicine known as humorism, and it would continue to be the foundation of medicine for another six hundred years.

The paradigm of the four humors in the field of medicine is first found in the works of Aristotle and then in the works of Hippocrates, who is known today as the father of modern medicine. The theory posited that humans are composed of four liquids, or humors, and that illness arises when these liquids are out of balance. The belief in the four humors was based in the physical evidence that could be found in dried blood. It was observed that when blood was left to dry, it would separate into four substances, which were labeled as black bile, yellow bile, phlegm, and . . . blood.

When the winter months cooled your humors, it was believed that it caused you to "catch a cold." To this day, many people still believe being cold causes illness, and we still use this phrasing to describe the conditions brought on by catching a rhinovirus or a coronavirus. If you were depressed, it was said that you had too much black bile, making you "melancholic." A person whose complexion was considered to be dominated by blood was said to have a "sanguine disposition," while people who were dominated by yellow bile were just bitter and rude. People who were dominated by black bile were likely to be lazy, and those who were dominated by phlegm were likely to be forgetful.

It was Galen of Pergamon (129–216 CE) who was widely credited as one of the greatest medical researchers of antiquity and made perhaps the greatest contributions in the proliferation of the medical practice of humorism, including the wide use of bloodletting. In Galen's time, menstruation was believed to be a way for the body to rid itself of bad humors, so it naturally followed that bloodletting would have a similar result. Galen was well respected, a physician to the Roman emperor, well-funded, eager to help people, and a prolific writer.

Galen's writings on bloodletting impacted the world of medicine for over a thousand years. In addition to physicians, he trained barbers in the art of bloodletting, which is still reflected in the red and white barber pole today, the red representing blood and the white representing a tourniquet. Galen developed a method of bloodletting based on the patient's age, disposition, the weather, the season, and the location.

The belief that humans are composed of four liquids, which determined their health and disposition, dominated the way humans saw themselves from the time of Hippocrates (circa 460–370 BCE) to the advent of germ theory in the 1850s. If we had been born and lived in these days, the four humors would have been as fundamental in our understanding of ourselves as anything that we base our knowledge on today. Everything from our health to our mood would have been interpreted as the balance or imbalance of these four liquids.

The history of the humors is long and far more complex than what is represented here. However, it should serve as a reminder that we base much of our beliefs and actions on misconceptions, and these misconceptions often become so foundational that they become a paradigm from which we cannot imagine an alternative. For over two thousand years, we just took it as a given that we were composed of four liquids, and this view was the starting point from which we interpreted our mental and physical health and well-being. Even our language still bears the mark of this paradigm that seems so ridiculous to us in the twenty-first century; however, it would feel strange to say that you caught a rhinovirus instead of saying "I caught a cold," wouldn't it?

The Mind-Body Paradigm

Any kid from the 1990s and beyond has heard of the *Teenage Mutant Ninja Turtles,* a show that had kids like me hoping to somehow be exposed to nuclear waste (in a good way?) all through our early adolescent years.

The Ninja Turtles cartoon told the story of four turtles who were once normal turtles, but when they were exposed to a mysterious nuclear waste, they were transformed into muscle-bound humanlike turtles. They lived in the sewers of New York City and fought crime. As a young boy, I just assumed that if I were exposed to this radioactive material, I would turn into a turtle and have a blissful life of crime-fighting, like the turtles on the screen.

The Ninja Turtles had two major enemies that they battled in every episode; Shredder, an evil ninja who was constantly trying to take over the city, and his boss, Krang. Krang was a disembodied brain from Dimension X. This disembodied brain used a robot body to move around while attempting to pull off a heist or take over the world.

If you are like most people, you probably believe you are much like the fictional Ninja Turtles bad guy, a mind that drives around a body, an operator of a robot that is much like other machines we drive around. It requires maintenance. It consumes fuel. It gets worn down over time. And like all machines, it breaks down. In many cases, we might look at our body and think to ourselves, "Wow, I must have gotten a defective unit!"

Our bodies provide us with a method of transportation and a way to interact with the physical world around us. The common misconception, however, is that we *are* the mind, and we *have* a body. We seem to believe that they are two different things; one is the master over the other. This concept is so embedded in our culture that it has shaped the very language we use in describing ourselves. This is at the heart of the concept of "mind-body."

The Geographical Divide

The separation of the mind and body can be seen in most ancient cultures. While the Greeks were champions of physical strength and skill, they saw the mind and the body as distinctly different things, and it is here that we see the beginnings of the modern idea that the two things are not only completely different, but they are in opposition to each other.

The philosopher Aristotle, in his proposed education system detailed in his major work *Politics,* declared that intellectual and physical training should never be done in the same year, "because the intellect and the body must not be worked hard at the same time, since the two kinds of exercise naturally counteract one another, exertion of the body being an impediment to the intellect, and exertion of the intellect an impediment to the body."[1]

This notion of the body as something that is opposed to the well-being of the mind can also be seen in much of the religious writings that followed. The body, often referred to as "the flesh," was seen to be something that needed to be constantly controlled, a hedonistic animal. We were called to be the masters of our bodily urges rather than letting our bodies lead us into sin. It is as if our minds and our bodies are separate entities with separate agendas, completely divorced from each other.

However, it was René Descartes in the seventeenth century who codified what we now refer to as "mind-body dualism." He is the philosopher most famous for proving his own existence by using his conscious thinking as his evidence, offering the often quoted example of circular reasoning, "I think therefore I am." Descartes determined that since the mind was, in his view, indivisible, and the body could be divided into parts, the two things were fundamentally different. It was also around this time that the body began to be viewed as a machine. Descartes stated, "I suppose the body to be nothing but a statue or machine made of earth."[2]

The mind-body paradigm has evolved over time, but the view still permeates our view of ourselves. Modern iterations of this view have evolved to view the parts of you that are below your neck as something that can be of good service to the mind if well cared for, kind of like a Buick. It is based in a particular way of seeing what we are, and what we believe about ourselves affects how we treat ourselves.

The Problem with the Mind-Body Paradigm

Like Descartes, we often see ourselves as operators of a body that is something other than us. We view ourselves from the neck down much like a machine, and we tend to treat ourselves accordingly. A machine can sit in one position in a small poorly ventilated space for eight hours per day without suffering injury. A machine has no feelings, no passions, no desires. Quite simply, a machine is lifeless and can only do what it is commanded to do.

When we believed we were composed of four humors, it made perfect sense to treat rheumatism with a rooster or to bleed a patient's illness out of them. But when we realized we were basing our actions on a misconception, we decided to look at ourselves differently and treat illness in a more effective way. The same thing needs to happen now with our conception of what we are. Are we an operator riding around in a flesh robot, or should we change the way we see ourselves?

Introducing You to You

What we have called the mind-body is one thing. A human is 37.2 trillion cells working together for the goal of surviving and thriving in the changing and varied climates of the planet Earth. And it doesn't all happen without an incredible innate intelligence that we often overlook and take for granted. At every level, there is an intelligence within you, and that intelligence is not something other than you, like a robot or a computer program. It is as much you as your conscious, thinking self who is reading this book.

The Innate Intelligence within You

In fact, the ease with which you read the words on this page is the result of the interwoven nature of what you are as a human. The same intelligence that assists your conscious experience of deciphering language with ease is orchestrating the symphony of information and matter that is you. Organs such as the stomach are digesting, veins and arteries are dilating or constricting, the kidneys are filtering, the blood is moving, gases are being traded with the environment; these are quite literally the physical expressions of your unconscious intelligence that you use to help keep all of you surviving and thriving. This doesn't begin or end at the neck. It's all you.

As you read this book, your diaphragm and intercostal muscles are moving to create negative pressure in your lungs, to invite fresh air into your lungs, and to facilitate a gas exchange with the outside air, which will be brought into your bloodstream, picked up by red blood cells, and moved through sixty thousand miles of intricately coordinated blood vessels via the beating of your heart. Your body will determine the speed and the volume of each beat with regard to the apparent needs of the rest of the organs and the apparent state of the whole organism relative to threats outside the skin, as informed by the sense organs that can be made to be more or less sensitive based on the intuitions of your predictive and reactive brain. All these processes and more are constantly happening and are constantly adjusted and modulated by unconscious messages that are being sent throughout your organism to improve your ability to thrive and survive on planet Earth. All of that is you.

The Conscious and Unconscious You

Rene Descartes believed that the mind is indivisible, but he was wrong. Cognitive research now shows that 95 percent of brain activity is unconscious, leaving only 5 percent as what we are consciously aware of.[3] Everything, from your heart rate to your emotions, from your personality to your digestion, from your hormone levels to your cognitive biases, from your creativity to your beliefs and values, is constantly being expressed by your unconscious-self.[4] It's not someone else. It's you. You are operating consciously and unconsciously to create and sustain your life.

Your conscious-self, which is the part of you that we have traditionally identified as "the mind," simply could not function without your unconscious-self. It is estimated that our senses are reporting approximately eleven million pieces of information at any given time. However, you can only consciously process approximately forty pieces of information per second.[5] The spare information, however, does not go to waste. All the information that your senses pick up is processed, interpreted unconsciously, used to make adaptive physiological changes, and, when your unconscious-self determines a need, it brings this information to your conscious awareness.

And this never stops. While you are sleeping, while you are eating, while you are in crowded rooms, you are never not receiving information from the outside world, and you are never not using that information to determine your safety status, your position in space, your position within social hierarchies, and all the other elements that your unconscious-self deems to be important.[6]

Just think of the last time you were at a social gathering. While you might have made a conscious choice of where to stand or when to walk to that part of the room, your unconscious-self had a lot to say about the situation, and it influenced your movements, postures, and behaviors with every step you took. When you saw someone who you wanted to talk to, you didn't have to consciously process who that person was or why you wanted to talk to that person; you just knew. Thank you, unconscious-self! And when you and your friend began to have a conversation, your unconscious-self filtered out all the other voices in the room to ensure that you could be engaged. But wait—someone just said your name in a conversation a few feet away. Were you consciously listening to that conversation too? Or did your unconscious-self monitor all of the voices in hearing distance and then filter them, only providing the conscious-self with awareness of the other conversation when the unconscious-self deemed it of value? While science still debates on where exactly in the brain this filtering occurs, there is a consensus that this happens at the unconscious level.[7]

The unconscious part of ourselves is always there to help us, and it doesn't begin or end at the neck. Let's do an experiment. Close your eyes, then hold up three fingers on your right hand and raise it above your head. Could you do that? Before you opened your eyes, did you know that you were successful? While much of this action was done with conscious control, it could not have been done without using unconscious processing and sensing, specifically using your sense of proprioception, the unconscious sense that allows us to determine our body's position in 3-D space. The unconscious side of you is quite literally embedded within your physical form. There is nowhere within you where you are not.

A Relationship with Ourselves and the World around Us

To be human is a never-ending relationship between our unconscious- and conscious-selves and the environment in which we find ourselves. Much of our troubles in the modern age comes from a lack of awareness of these foundational relationships, and this is widely because we treat ourselves like mind-body machine operators rather than whole beings. Modern humans suffer from disconnection—disconnection from within and from the environment around us—and this comes from a general misconception about what we are. We are organisms who exist in relationships with ourselves and our environment. We are not robot operators. And how we view ourselves affects how we treat ourselves.

2

Action Is
the Strategy

Have you ever looked at a tree and thought that maybe it is the more evolved creature? Trees aren't fighting wars or arguing in traffic. Nope. They're super chill. They even figured out how to make food out of, wait for it . . . sunshine. Seriously, plants are incredible. They seem to be able to grow just about anywhere, and some of them can live for hundreds or even thousands of years.

Of course, as often as we might ponder the superiority of plants, they have made a survival strategy based on the assumption that food will come to them and that the environment from which they sprouted will remain relatively unchanged. If the rains don't come, if something blocks their sunshine, or if the terrain shifts in a significant way, the strategy fails.

Our species employs a different strategy, one based on taking action. This is essential for understanding ourselves. We are built to be action-oriented. We must take actions within the environment to find food, avoid danger, and build prosperity. This action-oriented relationship with our environment is foundational to life as a human being, and we have developed a complex and powerful way of navigating and adapting to ensure survival and our ability to thrive on planet Earth.

Machines can sit in one place and fulfill their functions. So can trees. A human is not like this. Within each of us is a conscious and unconscious team working together to take actions in relationship with the world around us. For a moment, let's examine how the conscious-you and the unconscious-you once worked very naturally together.

A Day in the Life

There was a time when there were only two professions: hunter and gatherer. For most of human history, we have been hunters and gatherers, living in the natural environment for which we were built. For a moment, let's pretend we live in the earliest days of human history. What would life be like, and what would the roles of the conscious-self and unconscious-self look like, on an average day?

In this particular fiction, you find yourself waking up to the morning sunshine just peeking over the horizon. You just experienced a great night's sleep, full of deep recuperative sleep and dreams. You felt safe enough to go to sleep last night, which is a very vulnerable state in which to be if not in a safe place, because without your being consciously aware, your unconscious-self made sure to direct your conscious thoughts toward actions to eliminate potential threats. This was facilitated by the motivational network of your brain, using the neurotransmitter dopamine.

Dopamine is a neurotransmitter that acts as a reward chemical; however, contradictory to what many believe about dopamine, we do not get the "dopamine hit" after we do a task. We get it before. Dopamine is a neurotransmitter that encourages us to take actions to explore our environment and eliminate uncertainty. It is a major driver of actions that move us to discover new resources and eliminate possible dangers. It is what led us to check for snakes and other dangers that might be hiding so we can be sure that we are safe enough to change our state from waking to sleeping.

As you look around your surroundings, your eyes come across a long slender form. This is when your unconscious and conscious team goes to work. Note that, while we might be referring to the conscious-self and the unconscious-self in a way that makes them seem separate, it is to illustrate how these two aspects of you work together. You are as much one as the other.

Your unconscious-self is incredibly fast, and it can process incredible amounts of complex information seemingly instantaneously. It learns patterns quickly and can do complex thinking far faster than your conscious-self. This makes it a very valuable teammate. It scans the perimeter, picking up on the long slender object and makes the hasty interpretation: "snake!" In anticipation of a dangerous situation, it activates the fight-or-flight response within your autonomic nervous system and sends a powerful emotion, fear, to your conscious awareness. As a result, you become consciously aware of the potential threat, causing you to stop in your tracks and focus on the direction of the potential danger.

But your unconscious-self isn't done. By activating the autonomic nervous system, your unconscious-self changes the way your physiology is expressed, moving blood from organs such as your stomach and genitals to your legs and arms, preparing them for action. Your unconscious-self raises your heart rate, increases your breathing rate, and floods your blood with stress hormones. Your unconscious-self even enhances your sight, your sense of smell, and your sense of hearing to improve your ability to determine the level of threat that you may face. All of this happens without your conscious-self having to divert any of its attention, allowing the conscious-self to think critically about what it is seeing to find out whether it is a snake.

Your unconscious-self is incredibly fast and incredibly intelligent. However, it tends to jump to conclusions, and it tends to skew interpretation toward the negative. This is because your unconscious-self is not necessarily concerned with being right; it is trying to help you survive and thrive. If the long slender figure is a snake, it is to your advantage to react as quickly as possible and with an appropriate fear response. However, if it is not a snake, there is nothing lost but your calm.

Your conscious-self is slower, but it has the ability to check for accuracy. Yes, your unconscious-self can run circles around your conscious-self with regard to speed. However, it is not until your conscious-self takes a moment to examine the long slender figure in the distance that you realize that it is not a snake after all. It is a piece of vine that must have fallen out of a tree. Using your conscious-self's power of close examination and reason, you realize that this was a false alarm, that the fear that you feel is misplaced, and that you do not need to maintain a heightened state of autonomic arousal.

Of course, you don't consciously think these things, but now that your conscious and unconscious selves have worked together to solve the problem, your unconscious-self slowly returns your physiological and emotional state to relaxed and ready for bed. Your senses become dulled, your heart rate slows down, your hormones shift to encourage a good night's sleep, and once you have satisfied your unconscious-self that your area is safe for sleeping, your unconscious-self turns down the dopamine along with the other chemical messengers that make you alert. When this happens, your drive to explore the area to uncover any potential threats subsides, and you find a comfortable place to sleep.

✦ ✦ ✦

Now that morning has arrived, you must go to work, and your conscious and unconscious team is really good at being a hunter and gatherer. As you leave your safe place in search of a meal, your unconscious-self begins finding patterns in the approximately ten million pieces of information received by your eyes every second. After a life of hunting and gathering, your unconscious-self has become good at helping you sort out all of this information, sending "gut feelings" to your conscious-self about where to look for food and where to avoid. Assuming your unconscious-self has learned well, this is a huge help to your ability to thrive.

As the unconscious-self continues to scan the environment, it notices that the temperature has increased and takes measures to cool down. Constantly checking in with the hypothalamus, the unconscious-self uses the skin to help regulate the internal body temperature, opening and closing its pores to preserve or vent body heat, and if needed, releasing some of the body's water to cool the body by taking advantage of one of the properties of thermodynamics that creates a cooling effect when water evaporates.

All the while, your conscious-self is doing something that your unconscious-self cannot do: planning for the future. Consciously, you begin planning what actions you will take after the hunt is over. This forward thinking brings with it many unknowns. However, you know that if you do not save food for the coming season, you stand a great chance of starving. This uncertainty bothers your unconscious-self, which begins to add dopamine to the brain to encourage you to take actions to solve this problem and eliminate this uncertainty. You begin to ruminate on the problem, and your conscious attention becomes distracted from the hunt.

Fortunately, your unconscious-self is always there watching and observing the environment, looking for cues. When it identifies a pattern that it believes might be a suitable meal, it alerts the conscious-self, breaking you out of your rumination just in time to stalk your prey. The autonomic nervous system becomes activated, changing your physical expression to optimize your chances of success in the hunt, and your conscious and unconscious team go to work. Most of what follows is driven by your unconscious-self. Later your ancestors will call this the feeling of being "in the zone." While your autonomic state is once again fight or flight, you are not afraid. You are happy that you are getting the opportunity to get a meal. You are consciously aiming your spear and making some of the decisions involved, but when it comes to this part of the hunt, the more you let your unconscious-self take over and the less overthinking you do, the more intuitive and effortless each movement becomes.

After your successful hunt, you feel very happy. Your unconscious-self is pleased with the team, and so is your conscious-self. Together, you navigate your way back to safety, stopping only when your unconscious-self picks up a potential danger, sending awareness to the conscious-self to carefully examine, and picking back up again when you determine the path is safe.

When you arrive back to safety, your unconscious-self scans the environment, determines that you are safe, and engages the "rest and digest" function of your autonomic nervous system, changing your physical expression to suit the situation. Blood from your muscles returns to your digestive organs in anticipation of the meal to come. Your senses dull, your heart rate reduces, your breathing becomes slow and steady; your physical expression changes to recover from any injuries you experienced throughout the day, building muscle where needed, and repairing tissue.

It is at this time that you might have met someone special in your tribe who your unconscious-self approves of and therefore sends you amorous feelings about, encouraging you to form a bond. Deeming your environment to be safe, your unconscious-self has returned blood back from your skeletal muscles to your reproductive organs. And tonight might be the perfect night to use them.

This was how our conscious and unconscious team worked together for thousands of years; the unconscious-self is always trying to put us in the right state to take actions that will help us thrive, depending on the situation and the environment.

Fast-Forward to Today

Today, our lives are nothing like the ones our ancestors lived. We tend to look at ourselves mechanically, separating ourselves into parts, just like we are machines, disconnecting ourselves from the whole organism that we are. At the same time, we seem to have also grown roots like trees, living in environments that we cannot interact with as we once did. This leaves our team, which was built on taking action, in an awkward state of inaction. Your unconscious-self is still trying to assist the team to take action to survive and thrive, but in the modern context with our modern misconceptions about ourselves, we misunderstand what our unconscious-self is trying to do for us. So, rather than our unconscious-self and conscious-self acting as a team, we begin to believe that our machine is malfunctioning. We misinterpret the messages from our unconscious-self as symptoms of a broken machine rather than an attempt by a teammate to assist us in taking action.

While our unconscious-self can process incredible amounts of information with stunning ease, it still sounds the alarms at modern-day vines, thinking that they are snakes. Adding to the confusion, we have traded the potential threats of our natural habitat for an infinite number of potential threats that we can learn about on our tablets and smart devices. While many of these threats can be acted on, today we live in an interconnected global community, the size of which is nearly impossible to fathom and the implications of which are equally full of uncertainty. This leaves our unconscious-self screaming to take action even though, consciously, we know that nothing can be done.

The modern child is growing up in a world where we face threats that we cannot detect with our senses; a global pandemic, climate change, and the economic underpinnings of the world are like invisible snakes adding a seemingly infinite multiplier to the long list of all the uncertainties we face. Our eyes are glued to news, social media, and other sources of information, encouraged by our unconscious-self's steady stream of dopamine, as it is only trying to help us to take action to eliminate the uncertainty and possible threats.

Unlike the environment for which your unconscious-self was built, these modern problems cannot always be solved by simply examining a vine to find out if it is a snake or not. But your unconscious-self still does what it believes is in your best interest. It activates your sympathetic nervous system, it releases dopamine, and it releases norepinephrine from your locus coeruleus. This heightens your senses, which would be great if you were on a hunt. But most often we are lying in bed wishing we could go to sleep. Your unconscious-self is saying "Let's take action!" But your conscious-self knows that you cannot take action. This is a common disconnection within us that we experience as anxiety.

Rather than checking our bedroom for snakes, we check our phones every night before going to bed, and there is really no end to the potential snakes there. Eventually, we feel so tired that we put the phones down, maybe checking them one last time, then we close our eyes and try to sleep. But for many of us, sleep is hard to come by, and when we finally do get to sleep, we don't get the rest that we really need. When we wake up, we reach for our phones immediately and then drift to the kitchen to our life-giving coffee pot, where we caffeinate ourselves to a semblance of wakefulness. Then we get into a giant metal object and move at great speeds in high levels of traffic to our workplace and cram ourselves into offices and factories, much like a machine but a far cry from the human organism that lived as a hunter-gatherer for much of its history.

Perhaps the cruelest joke of the modern age is a concept called "the lunch break." This is when we expect our machine bodies to digest food on command without any regard for the events that have led up to this meal. Of course, the reality is that the unconscious-you, always trying to help you take action to survive, has activated your sympathetic nervous system due to the accumulated unchecked stress from your day. This shuts down your digestive organs to provide blood to your skeletal muscles in the attempt to give you strength to outrun whatever is threatening you.

What is worse is that since your stress hormones have been active all day, the salad that you swore you would eat for lunch just will not satisfy. No, your unconscious-self, believing that you must be in some kind of snake-filled hellscape due to the amounts of stress you have been experiencing, has been producing a steady stream of cortisol. This makes you crave quick energy sources like fats and simple carbohydrates. Cheeseburgers! French fries! Let's get drive-through! Of course, even if the drive-through food was nutritionally dense, in this state, your digestive organs are in no working order to digest it. Today there is an antacid empire built on this disconnection between humans' conscious and unconscious motivations.

Cortisol is a primary stress hormone that quickly increases blood glucose to supply your tissues with much-needed fuel. In short bursts, cortisol improves immune function and reduces inflammation. It is a beneficial stress hormone in short bursts where one experiences stress, and then when the stress subsides, so does the cortisol. However, in cases of chronic stress, one becomes used to having too much cortisol in the blood, which leads to more inflammation and a reduced immune function. While insulin reduces blood sugar, cortisol increases it. When our cortisol levels are left high, it can lead to a battle within ourselves to try to keep our blood sugar in a healthy range, which can lead to high blood sugar, weight gain, and type 2 diabetes. To make things even worse, there is also a correlation between high levels of cortisol and high blood pressure.[1]

When we consider the effect that stress has on our whole organism, it is no wonder that studies show that stress-induced inflammation is a common factor in most human diseases.[2] While modern living has led to many advancements that make our lives better, it seems to put us in a place of chronic unchecked stress that we desperately need to understand. This means understanding that our stress response is actually arising from a part of us that is trying to motivate us into action. Our lack of understanding about the fundamental nature of what we are as a species has perpetuated a disconnection within us that causes us to be unhealthy and poorly situated to thrive in our modern environment.

Oh, but our day isn't over yet. . . .

After we get out of work, maybe we have a hot date. I think there is a very underreported phenomenon growing in the developed world. The prevalence of Viagra and Cialis advertisements should give us a clue, and the fact that these products are now being packaged and marketed to younger adults should be telling as well. One of the most common complaints that I have heard from my clients over the years is that of low libido or sexual dysfunction. I've seen it in men and in women. Most of them don't tell me about it at first, but when I explain to them that being in a heightened state of stress will shut down sexual organs, they begin to share that they have had problems with intimacy and that maybe stress has had something to do with it.

While the prevalence of pornography has surely had an impact on young men and has been blamed for their impotence, I think we overlook the fact that chronic anxiety and unregulated stress also play a major role. When our unconscious-self believes that we are in danger, physical or psychological, it tries to help us by moving blood away from the sexual organs and reducing sex hormones. Whether we are carrying around stress from our day or simply afraid of not performing well, our unconscious-self can often hurt us while trying to help us. As the population of the world continues to rise, we are seeing a strange depopulation in many modern countries. While there may be many factors responsible for this, I think we overlook the effects of being in a chronic stressed state.

Much of what we suffer from in the modern age is a misunderstanding about ourselves, what we are, and how our organism's survival plan is often at odds with our conceptions about ourselves. Our misconceptions about what we are and our modern environment have caused us to live like planted trees while we expect to operate like machines. Our misunderstanding of how we really work leaves us suffering from stress, having no idea that the stress response that is killing us is actually our own unconscious voice, trying to help us take action to escape the perceived potential threats that it detects around us every day. And it is this misunderstanding that leaves us suffering from stress, unable to decipher our stress responses, and unaware of our unconscious voice acting to escape perceived threats daily.

This leaves us in a poor state for conscious decision-making due to the trade-offs that we make for physical performance at the cost of cognitive function. We can all probably relate to how difficult it is to think critically when we are under high levels of stress, which makes taking positive action to improve our lives very difficult. It has been shown time and time again that critical thinking declines rapidly when under stress.[3]

What is even worse is that in many cases, even if we can think critically and come up with solid action plans, many of the things that cause our unconscious-self to induce a stressed state simply cannot be acted on. We can all relate to sleepless nights due to worries about the next day. And modern humans also need to recognize that what we focus on, whether it is news, social media, and so on, also gives our unconscious-selves plenty of reasons to activate a stressed state. We are a species whose survival plan has always been to take action, but the modern world has delivered a nearly endless number of things to worry about that we can do nothing about.

Lives of Quiet Desperation and Emotional Disconnection

Of course, we also have emotions. It is not uncommon to be unsure what to do with them. What purpose do they serve anyway? For many of us, we might wish we actually were a mind-body machine instead of what we are because at least machines don't have to be bothered by such confusing and intrusive emotions.

It is generally agreed on within the world of cognitive science that emotions do serve an important function: to mobilize you into an action or behavior that your unconscious-self believes will benefit your survival or your ability to thrive. When your unconscious-self has an opinion on something, it will inform you via emotions. These messages are powerful and complex; sometimes pleasurable, sometimes uncomfortable, and often difficult to understand.

Sadly, most of us go our entire lives unaware of what our unconscious-self is trying to tell us. To put this another way, we often live our entire lives in conflict with ourselves, without knowing what we want. Deep down, our unconscious-self knows what we want, but for whatever reason, we fail to listen, making conscious choices with our lives that conflict with our unconscious desires, wondering why we are so unhappy, even though we shouldn't be.

Do you think our species would have survived if our ancestors were too anxious to sleep, unable to digest their food, or unable to engage in the reproductive process? Do you think living life without connection to our emotional needs and desires sounds like a life you would like to live? It is time that we reconnect with what we really are. We are relationships in action. We are relationships within ourselves, and how we express ourselves physiologically depends on our perception of the actions we believe we should take in our environment.

The unconscious-self is composed of many systems that we can never directly access consciously. For many of these systems, there is no good reason to want to look under the hood. For instance, while it might be interesting to understand why you were able to decipher the expression "looking under the hood" without having to think about it consciously, accessing this system within your unconscious-self would serve very little obvious benefit. The unconscious-self does an amazing job at things that do not (at least for now) have any conflict with modern life.

However, we can learn to form a better relationship with our unconscious-selves in ways that will positively impact our lives, allowing us to form a positive relationship within ourselves even in the face of the many stressors of the modern age. We can even learn to decipher our emotions as well, learning to listen to what our unconscious-self has to say to better align ourselves with what we really want and learning to deal with our fears and traumas in a gentle and effective manner. We can learn to work with ourselves, not against ourselves, and we can realign with our survival strategy, to take actions to survive and thrive within our environment once again. And for those things in life for which we cannot take action, we can learn to speak to our unconscious-self to help it remain calm. How do we do this? As with any relationship, it all begins with communication.

While a codified language with verbs, nouns, and adjectives is most commonly what we think of when we use the word *language,* there are many other kinds of language we engage in just as commonly. Gestures are an efficient way to communicate, and they send messages so efficiently that we have started adding them to our written language in the form of emojis. While there are some holdouts, most of us have recognized the incredible communicative value in physical and facial expressions when it comes to sending information to one another. Humans have likely been "speaking" this non-verbal language longer than we have been using words.

To communicate is a constant process of trying to convey meaning as best we can while trying to infer meaning as best as we can. It's not always a perfect process; we often misinterpret what our partner is trying to tell us. However, in most cases, the better we get to know the people we are trying to communicate with, the more clearly we understand them. We get to know their sense of humor, the way they talk faster when they feel a certain way, and how they seem to take a long time to get to the point when they are really excited. If we choose to, we can get to know ourselves in much the same way, learning to become aware of what our unconscious-selves try to say and learning to use breathing as a reliable pathway to communicate back.

As we will learn in the following pages, communication using our breath is much like the way we communicate using any other language: it relies on tone, speed, inflection, elocution, and what is appropriate for the situation. As we work toward a more positive relationship with ourselves, we will learn to listen and speak in this language with clarity. This is the Language of Breath.

3

The Language
of Breath

How do we make a positive relationship within ourselves that will allow us to take positive actions when we can and help us not lose our sense of peace in the times we cannot? How do we know what actions we really want to take deep down so we can move in alignment with our true desires? Like any relationship, it requires communication, and the rest of this book is dedicated to learning how to speak and, most importantly, how to listen to a part of yourself that you might have just realized was there all along.

Your unconscious-self is you. It's not someone else. In this philosophy of breath and self-awareness, we often refer to the unconscious-self as your partner or your teammate, which can make it seem like someone else. It is difficult to discuss this aspect of ourselves due to the limitations of language. So, while we discuss the two sides of you, your conscious- and unconscious-selves, remember that while these parts of you have different natures, who you are depends on them both. We might consider the language of breath as a system of learning to communicate with our unconscious-selves, but this is just another way of saying that we will learn to align the conscious and unconscious aspects of our selves. The way we frame it in this book helps us to contextualize and internalize this interaction so we can begin to take part in the never-ending flurry of messages within us.

>>>>>THE SMILING BACK EXERCISE

We will begin with an exercise that will serve to help us personify our unconscious-self. Just remember that even though we are speaking to the unconscious-self, we are speaking to you. As you are reading, begin to picture your own smiling face looking back at you, just as if you are looking into a mirror.

Now imagine your smiling face saying, "Okay, conscious-me, this is the unconscious-you speaking. I'm always here, trying to make sure that we are prepared for whatever the outside world is going to throw at us. I'll keep tabs on things and let you know what we need to worry about; I'll alert you to threats, patterns, and anything else that you're going to need to know about so you can examine things more closely, make plans, and use those amazing reasoning skills you have. Now, let's take positive actions to improve our life! Go team!"

Now, close your eyes and take a little time to introduce yourself to yourself. This is important for two reasons: One, this exercise helps you to see your unconscious-self as a partner. The second reason to do this exercise (and do it often) is to break down your old, internalized geography paradigm of mind-body, as if your essence were above your neck and your robot were below the neck. Embrace the fact that you are all of you, and all of you is working together to create who you are in relationship with your environment.

The Smiling Back Exercise is a great way to begin any breathing technique or session that we will cover in the rest of this book, and it is a good thing to remember any time you are experiencing feelings, emotions, and states of arousal. Let yourself visualize yourself smiling back at you, saying to you, "I'm always here, trying to help you to survive and thrive. I'm listening to you, and I'm always speaking to you, in hopes that my actions will help your actions."   <<<<<

Replacing "Mind-Body"

The mind-body paradigm persists, in many ways, because it is ingrained into our language, just like "catching a cold." Even though many of us have been trying to treat the human organism holistically for many years, we are left with words that reinforce the old paradigm. We need a new way to express the wholeness of the human organism, a word that we will use for the rest of this book.

Now that the introductions are out of the way, let's take one more step toward seeing ourselves as relationships. To do this we need to address the issue of language. All languages are sets of agreed-on symbols for concepts, items, actions, and so on. As we learn the language of breath, it is essential first to define some new key words before going any further.

Some Language about Language

philia (noun): The Greek word *philia* roughly translates to "affectionate non-romantic relationship" or "brotherly love." For instance, it is the root word for the city of Philadelphia, also known as "the city of brotherly love." It is ascribed to the highest form of love between friends, a relationship that might be seen among family members. What better way to refer to what we now know about ourselves? Within each of us is a relationship between our conscious- and unconscious-selves. Rather than focusing on "mind-body," we can simply focus on the whole human organism by using the word *philia*—a single word that symbolizes what we truly are: a relationship. Philia is all of you, your whole organism.

unconscious-self (noun): Everything intelligent within the philia that you do not directly access with conscious thought. This includes everything from proprioception to autonomic functions, from emotions to cell replication. Put simply, there is an incredible intelligence within each of us that depends on every other part of us to survive, and it knows what to do based on cues from within itself and outside itself. Sometimes it makes mistakes, and it often gets confused. But it is always trying to help the whole-you survive and thrive. This part of ourselves does not have the ability to use symbols like language, which is why we must infer what it is saying using the tools we will learn in this book.

conscious-self (noun): The conscious-self is the part of your philia that you access consciously. This includes everything from your conscious awareness to your voluntary muscle contractions, from your ability to reason to your ability to choose whether or not to act on the impulses of your unconscious-self. It can use symbolic representation that allows for the creation of language that we can use to attach meaning to emotions or other physiological phenomena.

What about the Physical Body?

Your physical form is the expression of the innate intelligence within you. All the atoms that make up our cells, organs, and tissues are manipulated and organized by an incredible intelligence that we have no conscious access to but that works to maintain life. We are not just pounds of flesh that are being moved around. Every part of what we are is intelligent and plays a role in making us who we are. How we express our physical form changes throughout our lives due to our relationships with the outer and inner world. There is no part of you that is not intelligent, and there is no part of you that is something other than you.

The Five Tenets of the Language of Breath Philosophy

1. Awareness is the foundation of all positive change.
2. Your unconscious-self is as much you as your conscious-self.
3. Your unconscious-self is always trying to help you survive and thrive.
4. The healthiest you is a whole self (philia).
5. Actions are the words.

Over the years I developed the Five Tenets as a way of encapsulating the essence of the Language of Breath Philosophy. In these five sentences, you get the core of the Language of Breath Philosophy, and it can serve as a reminder of the new paradigm we are entering. As we prepare to learn the language, let's take a moment to cover the foundations of this philosophy.

1. Awareness Is the Foundation of All Positive Change

There are many ways to become aware of your current physical state, and we have recognized most of them in the health and wellness world for quite some time. For instance, we can check people's body fat percentage, their bone density, their lean muscle mass; and we can test a person's range of motion, maximum lift, and a whole host of other things. We do this to establish baselines that we can use to determine progress. These are all ways of becoming aware. They allow for objective markers that we can refer to, measure, and compare over time.

These objective measurements are excellent, and they account for one level of awareness. However, subjective experience is also a powerful marker of awareness—one that we commonly overlook. No one other than you can know exactly how you feel, and this makes it difficult to explain—even to ourselves. We are limited by language.

When describing a subjective feeling, it is difficult to have objective measurements. We try to measure pain by using a numbered scale, but is a "7 out of 10" the same for me as it would be for you? Since the human experience is subjective, it is impossible to really know. For this reason, we have never developed a universal vocabulary for how we feel, and it is hard to think about things for which we have no vocabulary. And when things are difficult to do, we tend not to do them. So, while we might be able to say we are x number of years old and we weigh so many pounds, when we try to describe the way we feel, we often just say, "Fine . . . I guess." This lack of self-awareness ends now.

Many people have heard that the Inuit, who live in a terrain that is covered with snow for most of the year, have between forty and fifty words for snow, each of them describing a variation in the snow that falls. For instance, one word might describe slushy snow; another might describe dry flaky snow. Others might describe light snow, big puffs of snow, or sleet. This richness in the Inuit language's vocabulary for snow is an example of how humans tend to develop language to describe things that they engage with regularly.

As you practice building rapport with your unconscious-self, the most important part is allowing yourself to become aware of how you feel. This means engaging your conscious awareness as often as possible. Using the exercises in the next chapters, we will develop our subjective awareness using some objective measurements, but never forget that it is up to you to put in the effort to develop your sense of internal awareness, also known as the sense of interoception.

Interoception is the sense of internal awareness. There is a common misconception that humans have five senses: sight, hearing, taste, touch, and smell. However, this is not true. We have many more senses than this. For instance, we have the sense of proprioception to determine our position in three-dimensional space. If you close your eyes, for example, you know that you are upright. We also have another sense, the sense of interoception. It is the sense that we use when we determine that we are sick or nervous or upset. Essentially, this is the sense that we use when we need to answer the question How do I feel?

In the next chapter we will learn an exercise to help us develop this sense of internal awareness. Most of us have let this sense atrophy, but with practice we can become more aware of the state of our philia, allowing us to listen to our unconscious-self and infer what it is trying to tell us. When we do this, it allows us to work with our unconscious-self, rather than against it.

2. Your Unconscious-Self Is as Much You as Your Conscious-Self

We have already covered this topic in the previous chapter, so we won't discuss it much here other than to remember that we aren't talking to someone other than ourselves. Remember the old joke that it is okay to talk to yourself as long as you don't answer back? Well, we will be violating that rule when we use the language of breath. You will learn to "hear" what your unconscious-self is communicating by using your sense of interoception, and upon interpreting what that part of you is saying, you will be able to consciously send a message back, sometimes to say, "No, we aren't running from a bear," or perhaps to say, "Let's pick up the energy production," or "Let's balance all this energy so we can focus!" However, it is important to understand that all this communication is happening within you, so no matter what your unconscious-self is trying to tell you, it is coming from a place of love because it is quite literally a part of your philia that has your philia's best interest in mind.

3. Your Unconscious-Self Is Always Trying to Help You

Remember that our unconscious-self is very intelligent. It can process an incredible amount of information almost instantaneously, making sense of the world around us and endeavoring to help us to survive and thrive. However, while it is incredibly fast, it jumps to conclusions and can make mistakes. It can misinterpret the situation based on environmental cues. This can lead to uncomfortable emotions and incompatible physiological states for what we consciously desire to do. All of this can lead us to the misconception that our unconscious-self hates us or is working against us. This isn't true. This is all the more reason why we need to learn to create a positive relationship with our unconscious-self, and that requires understanding that even when it is making us feel uncomfortable or keeping us from getting sleep, it is doing that because it believes it is helping us.

4. The Healthiest You Is a Whole Self

When we learn to form a positive relationship within ourselves, we experience a wholeness that most people never feel, a level of self-knowledge and trust that leads to a happier and healthier life. When we can work as a team with our unconscious-selves, stressful situations become less daunting, digestion becomes less difficult, sleep more restful, and emotions less threatening. Most importantly, we can act with more confidence and poise.

When we see ourselves as a team, we can teach our unconscious-self to become a better partner while consciously becoming a better partner too. It takes time for this wholeness to manifest, so don't expect it to suddenly appear. This is a practice, not a performance. There is never a time when you will not be working on your relationship within yourself, just as you never stop working on a relationship you value with another person. The healthiest you is a team, and in time and with practice, you'll be able to trust your teammate in ways that you never thought possible.

5. Actions Are the Words

Cognitive science informs us that it is impossible to have direct conscious access to your unconscious-self. However, this does not mean that we cannot communicate. We do not have direct access to our friends or family, or any other person either, but we can still communicate with each other and form relationships. We do this by inferring meaning based on the information that our partner is able to share. We call this language. Communication is the act of inferring and transferring information, and we are a species that is action-oriented. This is the foundation of understanding what our unconscious-self is trying to say and how we can learn to speak to this side of ourselves with our breath.

We will be communicating using the action of conscious breathing, and we will be deciphering the actions of our unconscious-self using what we know about how it manifests changes in our physical expression. The manner in which we convey a message in any language affects its meaning, and it is no different in the language of breath. There are a nearly infinite number of ways to take a breath. Everything from the depth to the speed to the physical location of your breath will affect the messages that you send. This is much like the communications that we use in interpersonal conversations; our tone, presence, pace, inflection, and enunciation all shape the meaning as much or more than the words themselves. It is the same with how breathing speaks to our unconscious-self, and it is all because breathing is intimately connected with our nervous system in a way that offers a valuable pathway of communication to our unconscious-selves.

The unconscious-self also speaks using actions; however, because they are within us, we often overlook them, much to our detriment. We can decipher much of what it is trying to say using what we know about the actions it takes to change our physical and emotional state. We know that the unconscious-self is always trying to help us survive and thrive, and its actions—for example creating changes in heart rate, blood glucose, and sensory alertness—can be deciphered and interpreted, allowing us to be more self-aware, putting us in a place where we can respond using the language of breathing.

Language Lab 1

Now that we have defined some terms and covered the Five Tenets, it is time to learn to use the language of breath. After each chapter, there will be a language lab to help you develop your practice. The goal of these labs is to give you guidance, not to prescribe exactly how you construct your practice. Your philia, your environment, your life—they are specific to you. The only person who can truly decide how best to implement what you learn in each chapter is you.

For our first Language Lab, simply begin to try to think of yourself as a relationship. You are a relationship within yourself and in relationship with the environment around you. For this lab, simply try to embrace this new paradigm. Try to think of yourself as a whole being rather than a mind operating a body. Think about how you are in a relationship with your unconscious-self, who is always trying to help you survive and thrive on planet Earth. As you go about your day, or as you go about reading the next chapter, allow yourself to feel some awe at this incredible team that you embody.

4

Learn to Hear the Voice of Your Unconscious-Self

Most people approach breathwork in the old paradigm. They ask, "What is a technique for *xyz* problem?" They are searching for a code to input into their machine to get the machine to do the thing they want it to do—commands for their flesh robot. This is like learning to speak without planning to hear a reply.

I know how to ask someone "Where is the restroom?" in Spanish; however, as soon as they begin to offer me directions, I am left hoping they will simply point. I don't even know if they are giving me directions or telling me to get lost! To get value out of learning to speak, we have to be ready to decipher the reply. It is much the same with breathwork. However, people tend to learn a technique or two that is supposed to lead to a specified list of benefits (a.k.a. codes for their robot). In reality it's like learning to ask a question in a language you don't understand. Results will be limited!

Another thing that people will do is learn a breathing technique (again, for a specified list of benefits that they expect to plug into their flesh robot) and never practice it. Then one day, when they feel overwhelmed and flush with anxiety, they will try that breathwork technique they learned that is supposed to be good for this kind of thing. Again, results will be limited. Breathwork is not a code for your robot. It is a language. Like any language, it is full of nuance and takes patience and practice.

At first, it might sound like gibberish, but in time, you'll understand what your unconscious-self is trying to say. The next exercise will help us to become aware of the subtle language that we can learn to decipher when we apply our conscious awareness.

Learning the Skill of Interoception

Are you ready to hear the voice of the unconscious-you? Let's begin one of the most foundational exercises to your breath language training, the Interoception Exercise. This exercise is best practiced in a quiet place without distractions, especially early in your breathwork practice, but it can be practiced anywhere. If you have difficulty observing the voice of the unconscious-self, it helps to close your eyes and reduce as much sensory input from the outside world as possible. Yes, you can do this while reading this book, but try to remember the steps so you can do this on your own as often as you can, especially early in your breathwork practice. And for those who have been practicing breathwork for years, you need it too.

>>>>>THE INTEROCEPTION EXERCISE

Place your right hand over your heart and try to feel your heartbeat with your hand.

Can you feel it? It's there. Wait as long as you need to see if you can feel your chest's subtle movements in the palm of your hand. Without judgment, and without trying to make any sense of the language that you are observing right now, simply observe the pace of your heartbeat. Are you beating your heart in an even cadence? Is there a quickening or a slowing down? You are observing the very real "voice" of your unconscious-self, speaking to you in just one of its many channels of communication.

And that heartbeat? That's you! It's just another part of you, your unconscious-self, doing your best for the whole team that is the whole-you. Picture your own smiling face, smiling right at you, saying, "I've got this! I'll take care of the back of the store, and you take care of the front. Together, we will thrive on planet Earth!"

Now remove your hand from your heart. Place it on your lap, palm up, and focus on the palm of your hand. We are simply bringing our conscious awareness to the palm of the right hand.

Can you feel your heartbeat in the palm of your hand? It's there too! Can you bring your awareness to it? It has always been there. The subtle pulse of your blood, flowing through your veins and arteries. That's you. It's not just a mechanical device; it is a part of your philia that is working to provide all of you with the appropriate blood flow for the moment and for what your unconscious-self might be anticipating.

Now bring your awareness to the front of your right thumb. Can you feel your heartbeat just under your thumbprint? It's there too! And it has always been there. We are simply learning to become aware of it. If you don't feel it, take some time to try to focus. I promise you, your heart is pumping blood to your thumb right now. Some of us have just become so disconnected with ourselves that we have trouble separating all the information we are receiving. Just as when we first hear a new language, we are often unsure where one word ends and another begins, but with practice we catch on. Likewise, we can learn to decipher the messages of the unconscious-self. At first it might seem difficult. Don't worry. You will get it in time, with practice.

After you spend some time feeling your heartbeat in your thumb, move your conscious awareness down to your left leg. Focus your awareness on everything from your left buttock to the tips of your left toes. What do you feel there? Don't try to put it into words just yet. Just focus on feeling. We are focusing on building our awareness right now. Just feel. Stay here for at least thirty seconds, but feel free to focus on your left leg as long as you like.

Now bring your awareness to your left foot. Can you feel your heartbeat in your left foot? It's there too! And that's you. That subtle movement that you feel is your unconscious-self. It's just as much you as your conscious-self, but it's focused on keeping your philia safe and as successful as possible. Imagine your smiling face, looking back at you, smiling, as you focus your awareness on your heartbeat. "I'm taking care of us," your unconscious-self says. Maintain conscious awareness here for at least thirty seconds more.

Next, move your conscious awareness to your left big toe. Can you feel your unconscious-self here too? Maintain conscious awareness on your heartbeat in your big toe. You are observing a part of you that is just as much you as the part of you who is observing. Maintain focus on your left big toe for at least thirty seconds.

Let's have a challenge. Can you increase your conscious awareness? Maintain your awareness of your heartbeat in your left big toe, but now try to focus on your right big toe as well. Maintain your focus on the heartbeat in both of your big toes for at least thirty seconds.

Let's expand our conscious awareness even more. While maintaining your focus on the heartbeat in your big toes, can you expand your awareness to the heartbeat in your right and left thumbs? As this exercise gets more challenging, don't get frustrated. Self-awareness is a practice, not a performance. If you just can't seem to do this yet, be honest with yourself; you are adding to your interoceptive awareness, but you're also learning where your current limitations are. In time, you'll be amazed at how self-aware you'll be able to become. Now, if you can maintain this level of awareness, maintain it for at least thirty seconds before moving to the next step.

Now expand your awareness of your heartbeat to your feet and hands, maintaining awareness of your heartbeat for at least thirty seconds before moving to your arms and legs. Be sure that you can zero in on your heartbeat before moving on. As you detect your heartbeat, take time to observe it. Are your arms and legs all pulsing at the same time? Or is there a slight variance between their pulses? They are, after all, at different distances from your heart. Do you think this will make a difference? Does it? Maintain awareness of your heartbeat in your arms and legs.

As you maintain awareness of your heartbeat in your arms and legs, remind yourself that every heartbeat is determined by your unconscious-self, which is just as much you as the conscious-you who is observing it. We are becoming aware of our philia. Maintain this awareness and celebrate this with a smile.

As you smile, do you notice any change in the way you feel? Even if it is only the change in tension on your face, add this to your conscious awareness. However, it is likely that you experienced a slight change elsewhere, perhaps in a way that is difficult to describe. Don't worry about describing it right now, just become aware of it.

You're doing great.

Now, bring your conscious awareness to your whole self, every part of your self, from the tips of your fingers and toes to the top of your head. Can you feel your heartbeat? Can you trace the reverberations of each heartbeat throughout your philia? Where is the heartbeat the strongest? Where is it the faintest? Take your time with this. Spend at least thirty seconds observing.

Now make a frown. Does this change anything? Now make a smile. Does this change anything?

You might not have realized this, but this whole time, you've been breathing. Without you having to consciously do this, the unconscious-you took over. "I've got this," it said. "I see you are busy focusing on something! I will take care of us," this part of you said.

Now bring your awareness to your breath. Can you feel the cool air as it enters your nostrils? The warm moistened air as it leaves your nostrils? Just observe your breathing. Where is your breath going? What muscles are moving? Are you breathing quickly? Slowly? Just observe. No need to try to interpret these messages just yet. We are just becoming aware.

Repeat this exercise as many times as you like and take as long as you like. For many of us, this is the first time we have really listened to this language because, for most of us, we didn't realize that it was a language to begin with.

As you allow your awareness to come back into your regular frame, if you can, maintain at least a small level of awareness of the messages being sent by your unconscious-self. We are already beginning to build a better rapport with our unconscious-self simply by becoming more aware of its messages.

<<<<<

Relearning How to Feel

I worked with a police officer who spent many years working in the most violent areas of the city of Indianapolis. When I guided her through the Interoception Exercise, she said she had no trouble feeling her heartbeat in her chest, and even some in her hands, but when we got to her thumbs and toes, she couldn't feel a thing. She said she wondered if it was because she had learned how "not to feel" after years of seeing such heartbreaking and emotionally damaging things over the course of her career.

The fact is that many people from all walks of life commonly have difficulty with interoception, especially in the beginning. As we will learn later in this book, our experience of emotions is not an intellectual experience, it's a physical one. And when we don't understand where all of these sensations are coming from or what they are trying to tell us, they can be very distracting, scary, and even painful. As a result, many of us do our best to completely numb ourselves, atrophying our sense of interoception.

However, in time, and with practice, we can reclaim our internal sense of awareness, and when we do, we can learn to observe what our unconscious voice is trying to tell us. Today, the officer I mentioned is a certified trainer in a program I developed specifically for first responders. She eventually learned to feel her heartbeat in her thumbs and toes, and so can you. Just remember this if you struggled during this exercise.

Language Lab 2

> **Practice the Interoception Exercise at least once per day.**

You are taking your first steps in learning the language of breath! While you can continue to the next chapter if you like, to get the most out of your training, be sure to practice the Interoception Exercise at least once per day for the first week of your training. If you continue to read on before this week is done, that is fine. Soon you will learn the Awareness Exercise, which adds to the skills you will develop by practicing the Interoception Exercise.

Everything within the Language of Breath Philosophy is built on these exercises, and while many practitioners want to glaze over them, remember, this is how you build your ability to listen and understand the unconscious-self when it responds to what you will eventually learn to speak with your breath. Dedicate the time each day to developing your ability to cultivate your sense of internal awareness, and as you do, your fluency will grow far more quickly than if you ignore this foundational part of the practice.

5

The Rosetta Stone of the Language of Breath

To become fluent in any language, first we need a cipher—something that we can use to infer the meanings of the messages that we are being sent, and something we can use to encode messages that we want to send. The Rosetta Stone is an artifact that was found in 1799 by French military officer Pierre-François Bouchard during the Napoleonic campaign in Egypt. On it was inscribed a decree issued by King Ptolemy V Epiphanes in Memphis, Egypt, in 196 BCE. What set this discovery apart was that this decree was in three languages: Egyptian hieroglyphics, Egyptian Demotic, and Ancient Greek. Since it sent the same message in all three languages, it allowed scholars to decipher ancient Egyptian.

The Autonomic Nervous System

We also have a Rosetta Stone that we can use to decipher most of the language of our philia. It is our autonomic nervous system (ANS). It ensures that your heart is beating, your stomach is digesting, your lungs are breathing; it regulates your blood glucose, your stress hormones, your circulation, and everything else that naturally occurs without you having to consciously think about it.

This is all done without your conscious awareness. And that's a good thing! Imagine having to remember to beat your heart or having to consciously digest everything that you eat. You could never go to sleep because you would forget to beat your heart! Your unconscious-self takes care of this for you, and the autonomic nervous system is how it gets done.

SYMPATHETIC		PARASYMPATHETIC
HEIGHTENS SENSES	👁	DULLS SENSES
INHIBITS SALIVA FLOW		STIMULATES SALIVA FLOW
ACCELERATES HEART RATE	❤	SLOWS HEART RATE
INCREASES BLOOD FLOW TO MUSCLES		REDUCES BLOOD FLOW TO MUSCLES
INHIBITS STOMACH DIGESTION		MAINTAINS STOMACH DIGESTION
INHIBITS INTESTINES DIGESTION		MAINTAINS INTESTINAL DIGESTION
DECREASES BLOOD FLOW TO REPRODUCTIVE ORGANS		INCREASES BLOOD FLOW TO REPRODUCTIVE ORGANS

The ANS Rosetta Stone

As shown in the illustration, there are two primary branches of the autonomic nervous system, the sympathetic nervous system and the parasympathetic nervous system. These two branches correspond to your current state of autonomic arousal, which is informed by your unconscious-self's conception of the signals it is receiving. If your unconscious-self believes you are in danger or if it becomes excited or physically active, you become autonomically aroused, which leads you to become more sympathetic-dominant. If your unconscious-self believes you are in a safe and relaxed environment, you will become less aroused and become more parasympathetic-dominant. Your state of autonomic arousal will correspond with physiological changes that your unconscious-self believes will enable you to survive and thrive in the given situation that it perceives, and there are varying degrees of arousal that correspond with changes in your physiological expressions—your heartbeat, blood flow, hormones, and so on.

One of the strongest modes of communication from your unconscious-self is your autonomic state. It is a physical expression of what your unconscious-self is speaking, and it allows you to infer what it believes about the situation. When your heartbeat begins to quicken, your breathing becomes faster and more erratic, your mouth becomes dry, your digestion and sex drive shut down almost completely, and you might feel cold; these are all cues that the unconscious-self is gearing up for what it believes is a dangerous or an exciting situation.

The same can be said about the physiological messages we can observe when our unconscious-self believes we are safe and ready for rest. Our heartbeat begins to slow, our breathing becomes calm and relaxed, our digestive and sexual organs become more active, and we feel warmer as blood is diverted from the muscles to our organs.

The autonomic nervous system is a very useful cipher. It allows us to infer what our unconscious-self believes about what is happening or what is about to happen. Our unconscious-self is always processing information from our senses, running simulations, and observing patterns, and it makes real physiological changes to express what it believes the philia needs in a given moment. While we do not have conscious access to the unconscious-self, we can learn to listen to what it has to say by learning to become aware of our autonomic state.

This is our first major step in learning the language of our unconscious-self, which we need to understand before we can meaningfully speak back to it to form a positive relationship. We are quite literally learning a new language, and this can be challenging. However, it is something that can be done with practice.

Learning a New Language

If you have ever learned another language, you might know what it feels like to try to listen to a person speak in that language before you have any real grasp of it. My wife's family speaks fluent Spanish, and I have not mastered the language yet. This is primarily because I don't engage with it on a regular basis. They are very comfortable speaking English, and I think they just don't have the time to try to slow down their Spanish to help me learn. In other words, "Jesse, go take out the trash," is far easier for them to say than trying to say it in Spanish while pointing and gesturing to the trash can and then to the door. For me, hearing another language sounds almost the same as noise: there are so many sounds, inflections, tones, and cadences, and I have no conceptual reference for which they will make sense.

However, if you spend enough time learning a language, with regular practice and patience, you will find that the unintelligible sounds coming from the mouths of people speaking that language will eventually start to become less unintelligible. You start picking out a word or two. You can infer meaning from the person's gestures and tone. Over time, while you might not be incredibly fluent, you can understand when they ask you to take out the trash. And then, eventually, you might even start to feel confident enough to ask a question in that language or crack a joke. With regular practice, you become fluent. Eventually, you may even become so skilled at using the language that you understand how to use nuance and accent to add even more clarity to your messages. But, as all multilingual people will tell you, if you don't practice regularly, you'll start to lose much of the fluency that you earned. This is a perfect model for learning to use the ANS to decipher what your unconscious-self is trying to say.

Your unconscious-self is not going to slow down its messages to accommodate you. While some people will begin with a higher level of internal awareness than others, for most of us, we are receiving so many messages from our unconscious-selves that we don't even realize it is speaking at all. Therefore, to understand the unconscious-self's subtle messages we will be using the autonomic nervous system as our primary cipher, learning to become aware of its cues.

Heart Rate as a Cipher

Paying attention to our heart rate is one of the easiest ways to determine ANS activation. The faster your heart rate is, the more your unconscious-self is trying to help you take an action. A faster heart rate provides oxygen-rich blood to the tissues that your unconscious-self believes will need it most. A slight elevation in heart rate shows a slight activation of the sympathetic branch of the ANS. The faster your heart rate, the more assured you can be that your blood flow will be moved away from your digestive and sexual organs because your unconscious-self is preparing for a possible fight-or-flight situation. If your heart rate is closer to your resting rate, your unconscious-self is likely letting you know that it believes that you are safe and are possibly in a good place to eat, make love, or get some rest (the parasympathetic branch).

The heart rate is one of your most reliable ciphers for learning the language of your unconscious-self. The best way to get started with this cipher is to learn to accurately measure your heart rate. This can be as simple as finding your pulse and counting your heartbeats for a minute, but a more convenient way is to use a smart watch or a blood-pressure cuff. Once you have a reliable way to measure your heart rate, you can apply the following cipher:

1. Before you measure your heart rate, close your eyes and scan your philia, paying attention to your thoughts and any physical sensations that accompany them. Observe whether you, for example, feel hot, cold, anxious, relaxed, sweaty, or tense, and any other observations you can make about how you feel *before* you measure your heart rate.

2. Then measure your heart rate and begin to make the connection: "I feel like *x* when my heart rate is *x*." You are beginning to learn the language of your unconscious-self.

3. After you take your heart rate, think about what your heart rate says about your autonomic state. You now have an objective measurement (heart rate) that you can correlate to a subjective measurement (your body scan).

Learning a language means learning to make symbolic connections. In this case we are finding a symbolic relationship between our heart rate and how we feel emotionally and physically. Since your unconscious-self will never stop sending messages, it is important to measure your heart rate at different times of the day and when you notice changes in the way you feel. This helps us understand how the way we feel correlates to what the unconscious-self is trying to say.

A Sample Day

As you begin to learn the language of your unconscious-self, it helps to keep a journal or a record of your findings, especially for the first two or three weeks. Look for patterns and observe times when these patterns break down. Try to be open and don't make judgments. We are not trying to get a "good score." We are simply trying to learn about ourselves.

Use the previously listed steps daily during the following times. (This can be adjusted depending on your own personal schedule. I'm using what a standard day is for most people.)

Upon waking   This should provide you with your resting heart rate, which you can use as a baseline to compare to the rest of your measurements. This is the time that you are most likely in the most relaxed state. However, this might surprise you: Are you waking up in a state of anxiety or stress? Checking this rate regularly and comparing it with your subjective internal awareness can be quite revealing.

Before going to work   This is a common time to feel stressed because it is before the thing that normally stresses us out the most: work! Check in with your unconscious-self. What is it anticipating? How do you feel, and what heart rate corresponds?

Before eating lunch   This is a crucial time for our unconscious-self to become more relaxed so we can accept the nutrition we are about to ingest. If the unconscious-self believes we are in danger, our digestive organs will be shut down. In time, you will learn how to use your breathing to help assure your unconscious-self that it is okay to relax.

Midafternoon   A few hours after lunch, check back in, making correlations between the way you feel and your heart rate.

Before dinner   Again, is your unconscious-self ready for dinner?

Early evening   This is a good time to check in with yourself to see if your philia is on the same page. For most of us, this is a time when we are not at work, but we might be obsessing about work. What does your unconscious-self have to say during this time in your day?

Before bed Is your unconscious-self ready for a night of restful sleep, or is it running from a bear? This is a time to learn about what it believes about your well-being and safety.

Wildcard Anytime you experience a noticeable change in the way you feel, check in. First, congratulations for having a level of awareness that can identify a change! Secondly, let's learn from this noticeable change using the cipher.

The Simple Cipher

Simply put, the higher your heart rate is above your resting heart rate, the greater degree of autonomic arousal you are experiencing. This means that your unconscious-self is activating to put you into the best possible state to act. It is doing everything it can to support your philia in hopes that you will survive and thrive.

It is important to understand that ANS activation is not necessarily a bad thing. Again, we are not trying to use this cipher to judge ourselves. We are simply using it as an easy way to understand what the unconscious-self is saying at a given time.

A raised heart rate does not mean that you *should* feel a certain way. For instance, you might feel excited and content and find that your heart rate is high. Just remember that this is not binary code. Perhaps you are excited because you are going to sing a solo in front of a crowd or because you are surfing. These are also times when the unconscious-self knows that you will need added energy and autonomic arousal. Take note of this as well. Compare how you feel to your heart rate and make connections.

However, after checking in while using the heart rate as your cipher, you might notice that there is a disconnect between your conscious goals and the physiological state that your unconscious-self has put you in based on its interpretation of your situation.. This is common. Soon you will learn to take an active role in the never-ending conversation that is happening within you. For now, we are learning to become aware. Without awareness, anything we say would be either gibberish or worse—it could speak the opposite of what we mean to say!

Language Lab 3

> Practice the Interoception Exercise at least once per day.

> Practice using your heart rate as a cipher in the way discussed in this chapter.

This is an exciting time in your language learning. You are beginning to observe connections between your objective measurements and your subjective experiences, using heart rate as a cipher. However, you can also expand your use of ciphers to any of the other items listed in the ANS illustration. We often use the heart rate in the beginning because it tends to be a more objective measurement than trying to determine the activation of your digestive system or the rate of blood flow circulating in your skeletal muscles. However, if you observe any of the other shifts that we described in this chapter, take note. The more aware you can become of your internal state, the better.

As you continue your practice, especially for the next week or two, using the sample heart rate check-in times described in this chapter will help you get to know yourself better. I strongly recommend using a journal rather than simply trying to remember. Sometimes we miss patterns if we don't write things down. The goal is to become more aware of how your philia operates throughout the day by using these preselected times to make a conscious connection between your objective measurement and your subjective experience. Trust the process and watch your connection to your unconscious-self grow.

6

Your First Words

The language of breath is much like any other language: there are words and syntax, which convey meaning, but there is also much more to the language, such as situational appropriateness, inflection, and tone. We will begin with some words and syntax, but understand that if you don't feel that your unconscious-self understood the message, it might be because you need to learn the other elements of the language (which we will cover in the next chapters).

Phrase in English: "Let's calm down."

Phrase in the language of breath: the Extended Exhale Technique

We will begin with a phrase that is likely one that you will use the most. With time, you'll be able to speak this with clarity. Before we begin this first lesson, become aware of how you feel in this moment. Check your heart rate and practice making connections as we learned to do in the previous chapter. This will help you to know how appropriate it will be to say, "Calm down." Are you already calm? Or perhaps you need energy to do something. "Let's calm down" is only appropriate to say when you are more activated than what is appropriate for the moment.

So, if you are not already calm, this is a great time to learn this phrase. If you are calm, stop reading and do ten burpees. Yes, you read that right. Or perhaps you can move around or do some jumping jacks. This will tell your unconscious-self to activate. This will give you a great opportunity to send a signal that you should calm down again.

Saying "Let's Calm Down" in the Language of Breath

Sit up with proper posture and try to avoid distractions. We will discuss how things like posture and physical cues play a role in the tone and inflection of your messages in the next section, but for now, just try to sit up straight and avoid distraction. It is time to send a simple message.

1. Bring your awareness to your breathing, making no changes, just bringing your awareness to it.

2. Now take a deep inhalation through your nose, bringing your breath down to your lower abdomen and only filling your lungs to about 70 percent, starting at the bottom and filling up slowly.

3. Exhale as slowly as you can through your nose or your mouth. Keep the flow of air as even and consistent as possible. Make the exhale as long as you can without straining, and empty your lungs.

4. Repeat this for at least two minutes.

When you are done sending this message, you can either go back into natural breathing or you can continue to send the message, depending on how you feel. Now is the time to check in with your heart rate and scan your physical and emotional feelings.

If you noticed a reduction in your heart rate or if you feel more relaxed in general, you can rest assured that your unconscious-self received the message and interpreted it in the manner that you sent it. That is great! However, for many practitioners, results will be limited. This is for a few reasons.

One reason why you might have limited results is because you are inexperienced. Just like anyone learning a new language, you can't expect to speak with perfect clarity on your first try. It is likely that your unconscious-self hears you, but just like when we learn any new language, it is easy to stress the wrong syllable or put inflection in the wrong place. This can obfuscate the message that you intend to send. Be patient with yourself. With practice, you will see progress.

Also, you may have limited results with sending messages to your unconscious-self via a breathing technique because you are competing with messages coming from the environment. Remember that your unconscious-self is monitoring countless signals from every direction. While we can send messages to the unconscious-self, we must understand that it will be one of many messages that the unconscious-self is receiving. With time, we can learn to form a better relationship within ourselves so that our message is viewed with a greater level of importance, but at first, it can be just one more message in an ocean of messages, especially when we are in environments that have a lot of people, sounds, movement, and other "loud" messages.

A third reason why your message might not have been clearly received is that you were speaking with poor tone and inflection. With respect to using breathing as a language, this refers to all the physical actions that you performed in taking and releasing each breath. There are a lot of ways to take a breath! When you are given instructions like, "Take a deep inhalation through your nose, bringing your breath down to your lower abdomen and only filling your lungs to about 70 percent," this doesn't consider the seemingly infinite ways in which such an action could be done. In the next chapter we examine all the physical actions that are involved in taking each breath, what we will refer to as the "tone and inflection" of the messages that you send with each breath. But first, let's learn more about the Rosetta Stone of the language of breath.

Why Breathing Speaks

If you look at all of the things that are governed by the autonomic nervous system, you'll notice that nearly all of them are not things we can consciously access. Breathing, on the other hand, is something that we take turns with between our conscious- and unconscious-selves. When we take our conscious awareness off breathing, the unconscious says, "Okay! I'll take over for now." And when we bring our conscious awareness to our breath, the unconscious-self begins to observe our breathing and listens to the messages that this controlled breathing sends.

This shared access to breathing offers us a communication pathway. You see, the unconscious-you is using the same Rosetta Stone as the conscious-you: the autonomic nervous system. Just as you can use the heart rate as a way to decipher what the unconscious-you believes about what is happening or what is about to happen, your unconscious-self will listen to your breathing to infer what you have to say too.

Let's do an easy test. Start breathing like you are running from a bear. Can you imagine how this might be? Heavy breathing, fast and full, allowing the chest to fill to the max, possibly using the mouth to breathe? Just sit there and breathe like that for a minute if you can stand it. When you are done, perform the Interoception Exercise that we learned earlier. Has your heart rate quickened? Do you feel a surge of energy? Perhaps you feel a change in temperature?

Only one thing changed when you decided to breathe like you were running from a bear, but because you changed your breathing to stress breathing, your unconscious-self received a message to become more sympathetic-dominant (stressed state). You spoke to the unconscious-self, and it replied. Congratulations! You are learning to use the Rosetta Stone of the ANS.

Fine-Tuning Your Cipher

While we will learn to send clearer and more nuanced messages using the language of breath, it can be helpful to understand a foundational principle of breathwork. Simply put, if you breathe like you are calm and relaxed, your unconscious-self will receive a message that things are safe and that you should become more relaxed. If you breathe like you are panicked and afraid, you'll send a message that you should activate to become more prepared for potential danger.

This raises the questions: What does relaxed breathing look like? What does it mean to breathe like we are calm? A simple way of looking at it might be to say that the faster and more erratic your breath, the more stress you are speaking to your unconscious-self. Slower and smoother breathing tends to be relaxed. When you were doing the "running from the bear" experiment earlier, you probably used your mouth and your chest to breathe. If you are reading a book or relaxing in a hammock, your chest is probably less active and your breathing more nasal. These are all cues that form a message.

However, we often inadvertently teach our unconscious-self bad habits, such as dysfunctional breathing, leading to a feedback loop from within your philia: the unconscious-self breathing in a stressed way that sends a stress message to the unconscious-self, which activates the sympathetic side of the ANS, leading to more stressed breathing, which, again, sends a stressed message to the unconscious-self. This can lead to chronic stress and anxiety. Many people live with this and don't realize it. When we take conscious control of our breathing, we can change the message.

The good news is that we don't always have to be in conscious control. If your goal is to be in control, you'll never be able to rest. We can form a trusting relationship with our unconscious-self, relearning on a conscious and unconscious level how to breathe calm and confidence with every breath. The next chapter covers tone and inflection, an area of communication that is commonly overlooked, especially within the breathwork world, because it's not only the words that carry meaning but also how you say them. ·

Language Lab 4

> Practice the Interoception Exercise at least once per day.
> Practice using your heart rate as a cipher in the way discussed in this chapter.
> Practice using the technique we learned in this chapter to let your unconscious-self know that your philia is safe and can calm down.

We are beginning to learn to speak and listen to the conversation within our philia. It is an exciting time in the learning process. However, don't forget to focus on growing your internal awareness by practicing the Interoception Exercise and by comparing your heart rate to your subjective feelings. Practicing these foundational skills will allow you to understand your unconscious-self more fully when you enter into more active dialog in the next chapter.

7

Learn Breath Mechanics

Regina was a 911 operator of over fifteen years. Each day she answered the phone, and on the other end was someone who was having the worst day of their life. Drug overdoses, suicides, rapes, break-ins, heart attacks; from the time she sat down to the time she went home, her job was to coordinate with the appropriate emergency services to keep victims calm, safe, and alive.

I met Regina at an annual retreat I lead specifically for those who work in the field of public safety. Like everyone else who had arrived at the retreat center, she often felt that she was unable to relax, always a little on edge, and never able to be fully happy. We know this as a state of chronic hypervigilance, and we see it frequently in the public safety world.

During these retreats and workshops, I teach functional breathing, which is what we will be covering in this chapter. The way we take each breath, the muscles we use, and the order in which we use them affect our nervous system in profound ways that can create a positive inner relationship, but when dysfunction creeps in, each breath can unknowingly create disharmony within our philia, exacerbating the stress we already experience from our environment.

After I led Regina's group in a functional breathing exercise, I asked the attendees to lie down and practice their breathing while my assistants and I went about the room, giving each person a hands-on assessment along with coaching in how to improve. When I got to Regina, she looked at me with eyes wide in astonishment.

"I don't think I can move my diaphragm at all," she told me.

Like most of the attendees, she had developed such a level of breathing dysfunction that she found it difficult to consciously activate her primary breathing muscles.

"I don't think I can either," said the officer lying next to Regina.

It was true: with each breath, their chests would rise, their necks would strain, their shoulders would hunch, but their tummies and their rib cages barely moved. Only in that moment did they realize that with every breath they were adding stress to their lives—stress that they had probably been suffering from for years. While this is common in nearly all high-stress careers, I have seen an especially high prevalence of this in the public-safety population. Everything from the hypervigilance required in their work to the pounds of tight-fitting gear that they must wear daily surely contributes to the poor breathing that I commonly witness when assessing them. Regina was sitting in a chair all day, unable to take physical actions to help the people she spoke to, empathetically responding to the desperation she surely heard on the phone.

I am happy to report that in only a few minutes, using what you will learn in this chapter, we were able to help Regina and the other first responders to improve their breathing, and after the retreat, practicing regularly, Regina and the others learned to speak calmness with every breath.

Within the Language of Breath Philosophy, the way you breathe affects the messages you send to your unconscious-self with each breath in much the same way as your tone and inflection affect the meaning of what you speak out loud.

Tone and Inflection

Tone and inflection are so foundational to communication that we usually never formally learn them even though they convey most of the message. Isn't that strange? With all our emphasis on spelling and typing, we tend to leave kids to learn the physical act of communication on their own. Of course, we all know that when we communicate, tone and inflection often convey more meaning than the actual words that we speak.

Consider the phrase "I love you." It's a powerful phrase. If it is said with a pleasant tone and consistent inflection, it might be received as a genuine message of affection. However, if you were to scream it while thumping your chest, it will likely be interpreted in a completely different way. While we don't normally make such major mistakes in tone and inflection in real life, one of the most common sources of friction in a relationship is a misinterpretation based on tone. There is a reason why anyone who is in a relationship long enough will likely say and hear the phrase "It's not what you said; it's how you said it."

When it comes to the language of breathing, it's not always the breathing technique that matters as much as how you breathe it. So how do we use proper tone and inflection when speaking the language of breathing? To learn this, we need to learn functional breathing.

The Physiological Act of Breathing

The act of breathing facilitates a gas exchange between the outside environment and your bloodstream with the primary goal of ingesting oxygen and releasing excess carbon dioxide. Oxygen absorbed in the lungs goes directly to the heart and is then pumped throughout the more than sixty thousand miles of your circulatory system, feeding every cell with the primary components for making cellular energy.

Each cell houses mitochondria that take the oxygen, and along with glucose, create cellular energy, also known as adenosine triphosphate (ATP). This is a process known as cellular respiration, and it is happening right now without you ever needing to be consciously aware of it. You do this unconsciously so that your conscious-self can focus on other things, like hunting, gathering, and thriving within your environment.

You might be surprised to know that your lungs are not mirror images of each other. Your right lung is slightly bigger than your left: your right lung has three lobes while your left only has two. This is to leave room for your heart. Just take a full inhale and see if you can feel the effect of the expansion of your lungs within your chest cavity. Can you feel below your lungs? You might notice a slight difference on your left and right sides as you explore the feeling of expanding your lungs downward. On your left side, you have your stomach, on your right side, your liver. If you recently ate a big meal, you would likely experience a different sensation than if you have an empty stomach.

Breathing with lungs involves the law of gases. A gas will always travel toward the area with the lowest pressure. When we open our lungs, we reduce the intrapulmonary pressure (pressure in our lungs), inviting the air to enter. The air passes through the sinuses, the pharynx, the trachea, the primary bronchi (right and left), the secondary bronchi, the tertiary bronchi, the bronchioles, and finally makes it to the hundreds of millions of alveoli that line the inside of each lung. If air doesn't make it to the alveoli, the gas exchange cannot occur. This process is facilitated by specific muscles that, when used as designed, allow for an appropriate gas exchange for any given situation.

However, no matter how much air makes it to each alveolus, it is only useful if there is blood available to carry the gases. If you think of an alveolus as a bus station, each breath might represent a potential group of bus riders, and red blood cells might represent buses. For an effective bus system to exist, one would want to put the greatest number of passengers where the maximum number of buses stop. The bus stops where fewer buses frequent might be used as an overflow in times of high demand. However, for the most part, one would likely want to maximize the efficiency of the bussing system as a whole. The same concept applies to breathing.

Our lungs can be broken into three sections based on ventilation (the amount of air that can enter an area) and blood perfusion (the amount of blood flow present in each area). Ventilation is mostly affected by the muscles and structures that are used in the act of breathing, and perfusion is largely affected by gravity.

The upper part of the lungs, which are largely above the heart, have larger alveoli, which are less effective at exchanging oxygen and carbon dioxide. This area of the lungs has very little blood flow, which means that it is the least efficient at facilitating gas exchange. Using our bus station analogy to understand the upper region of the lungs, this means there will be many passengers who will not be able to find a bus to ride.

The middle region of our lungs has smaller alveoli than the upper region, making them more efficient gas exchangers. There is also more blood present in this area, which means that when air is breathed into this portion of the lungs, more gas exchange occurs. In other words, there are more buses available for the passengers.

The lower lobes of the lungs house the smallest and most densely packed alveoli, which are the most efficient, and due to gravity, the lower lobes are also where there is the highest amount of blood flow. This means that when air makes it to this area, the potential for gas exchange is the highest. Using our bus station analogy again, there are so many buses available here that passengers will almost always get picked up.

Breathing involves creating a vacuum in the lungs that will guide air to each of these three areas depending on which muscles we use, and our unconscious-selves expect a specific order in the use of these muscles. This is much like how we generally expect a specific tone in someone's voice when having a conversation. When the tone matches what is being said, it enhances the meaning of the phrase. If the tone in the voice doesn't match what is expected, we tend to wonder if something is wrong. The same is true for breathing. How we utilize these three areas of our lungs informs our unconscious-selves about the current state of the philia, enhancing or obscuring the meaning behind the phrases we speak to our unconscious-selves when practicing breathwork techniques.

With very few exceptions, we are all born breathing with ideal breath mechanics, a product of the innate intelligence of our unconscious-selves. If you have ever watched babies breathe, you will observe that they breathe into their bellies, they don't breathe any faster than they need to, and they rarely seem stressed out. As they become more mobile, they look like little sumo wrestlers walking around, allowing their bellies to relax as they walk in their diapers. So many movements that will be difficult for them to perform later on seem easy for them. For example, a child under the age of two years can usually perform a perfect squat; their mobility has not been altered by sitting in chairs. The same is true for humans and breathing. In fact, a study conducted in 2022 tested 1,933 athletes from ages ten to twenty-five and found that 90 percent of them were breathing dysfunctionally.[1] This is especially telling since the individuals tested were relatively young, and athletes are generally the fittest among the population. It is a good reminder that breathing dysfunction is not rare and that we all need to be vigilant in improving and preserving our own.

Tone and Inflection = Presence

Babies are master breathers. They aren't practicing breathing techniques because they don't need to. They still have a great relationship within themselves. And just as it is within human interpersonal relationships, when the relationship is in harmony, simply being present is enough.

Have you ever seen friends who are so comfortable with each other that they can sit in silence? Maybe you are in a relationship like this: partners walking side by side in silence, completely comfortable with each other because they have established such a positive rapport. Much can be left unsaid because everything is said with each partner's presence.

We also observe a person's presence before we decide to get into a relationship. When people have an "off vibe" or seem to have an angry disposition, we tend to not want much to do with them. We can use this as a model for using our breathing to create a positive relationship within ourselves. We want to impart a presence of calm and reliability, and we do that by breathing like a baby.

Let's relearn how to breathe like we did when we were babies. This will help us to impart a solid presence within our philia. Before we relearn how to breathe, be prepared for this to feel a little weird. It is likely that you have been breathing improperly for most of your life. The process of correcting your breathing mechanics will take time and practice. And it will never be something that you don't have to practice. Every breath you take, whether it is conscious or unconscious, imparts a message, so how you take each breath matters a lot.

The Breath Wave

The muscles you use and the order in which they are used matter. Just as specific muscle patterns in your mouth create tones, syllables, and words, so do our breathing muscles when we're speaking the language of breath.

You might have heard that you should breathe with your diaphragm. Perhaps you have been told to breathe into your belly. While these instructions are not wrong, they can seem a bit ambiguous. In this section, we will learn how to use our breathing muscles to create the tone and presence that will create a positive relationship within our philia.

The term *the breath wave* describes what functional breathing looks like if you were to view yourself lying down from the side. It facilitates the fullest and most efficient breath, allowing for the most efficient gas exchange in every breath. It uses specific regions within your torso as markers to help provide guidance on where to "put" each breath. This section will provide you with some of the vocabulary that we will continue to use as we learn more about how to use our breathing to send messages.

Checking Your Current Breath Wave

Before we learn the functional breath wave, let's conduct a test to see what your current breath wave is like. Awareness is the foundation of all positive change, and it is important to become aware of your current breathing pattern to see what you need to work on first. What tone and presence are you currently bringing to your philia? Let's find out!

To get the best measurement, use the camera on your phone or laptop. A mirror is a poor tool for this kind of assessment because it gives you immediate feedback, which will likely influence your breathing, leading to an inaccurate test. For these assessments, just breathe in a way that feels normal to you.

ASSESSMENT 1

1. Empty your lungs as much as you can and take a slow big inhale to full lungs.

2. Repeat four times.

3. Give your camera a "thumbs up." You have completed the first assessment.

> **ASSESSMENT 2**
>
> 1. Breathe full breaths quickly (three seconds inhale, three seconds exhale) for about twenty seconds.
> 2. Give the camera a "thumbs up."

> **ASSESSMENT 3**
>
> 1. Breathe as fast and fully as you can for twenty seconds.
> 2. "Thumbs up" to the camera.

Assessment 1: Your focused breath wave

Assessment 2: Your fast and focused breath wave

Assessment 3: Your active breath wave

We test all three because there usually comes a point where even the most functional breather's breath wave will break down, which is another way we bring awareness to our practice.

When you have completed filming your current breathing pattern, keep it on file to compare it with the pattern that we will learn in this chapter. As you implement what you learn about functional breath mechanics, come back to this section and repeat this filming process to observe your progress.

Compare what you observe in your video with what is described in the next section and make regular efforts to make corrections as needed. Always remember: this is a practice, not a performance. If it were a performance, it might be appropriate to make judgments. But that isn't what this is. Breathing is something you will do for the rest of your life, so just remember that every breath can move you closer to better breathing. If this one wasn't great, the next one is a great opportunity to improve.

How to Breathe

The following graphic is a visual representation of the three major parts of the breath wave. This follows the path of the most efficient gas exchange within the lungs to the least efficient, maximizing each breath. A functional breath activates in the following order:

Inhales: belly → ribs → chest

Exhales: chest → ribs → belly

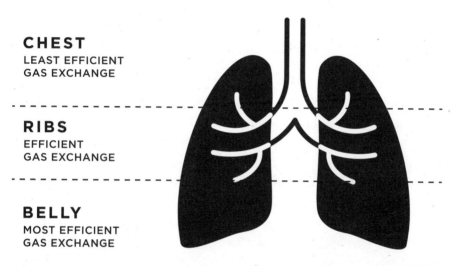

CHEST
LEAST EFFICIENT
GAS EXCHANGE

RIBS
EFFICIENT
GAS EXCHANGE

BELLY
MOST EFFICIENT
GAS EXCHANGE

The location of each breath adds tone and inflection to each breath, leading to a presence of calm and reliable or alert and shaken.

This does not mean that every breath should engage all three major parts of the breath wave. It is simply the order that your unconscious-self expects if you do engage all three. One should always follow the next; they should never be done out of order unless you are intentionally trying to add an unusual tone to your message. It is by using the three major areas of the breath wave that we add tone and inflection to the messages we send with breathing techniques.

However, as we discussed earlier, in a positive relationship, presence alone is important. When we learn to breathe functionally, we convey a calm and focused presence. The unconscious-you will pick up on that, and it will provide reassurance. This helps to build the positive rapport within our philia that leads to a strong team.

Within these major areas of the breath wave (belly, ribs, chest) there is nearly an infinite number of "stations" along the path of the breath wave.

That is to say, one does not just breathe into the belly. One can breathe a little bit into the belly, a little more than that, a little more than that, and so on until this region of the breath wave is full. One can breathe to the deepest part of the belly, or just activate the middle or upper part of the belly. In this way, how you take each breath is much like how you say a word or phrase.

Station 1: The "Belly"—Using the Diaphragm

Your diaphragm is one of your primary breathing muscles, and it should be the first muscle that you activate on every inhale and the last muscle you relax in every exhale. This will create expansion in the lower lobes of your lungs, inviting air to the part of your lungs that has the best capacity for gas exchange, as we just discussed. When the diaphragm contracts, it pulls the lower lobes down, reducing the pressure in this area specifically. In most situations in life, this is the only part of the breath wave that should be active, since the lower lobes are more than capable of facilitating a gas exchange for your needs. Your unconscious-self associates breathing that is low and slow with being calm and relaxed. Just think: if you are calm and relaxed, do you need to fill your lungs all the way to the chest? Of course not. We only do that when we are running from a bear or charging a hill. When we relax, we breathe slow and low, down in the belly, just like a happy pot-bellied baby.

We typically call this part of the breath wave, the "belly." Every breath you take should begin in the belly, but let's get even more specific by identifying the focal point where every breath should begin. To do this, follow these directions.

Finding the Beginning Point of Every Breath

1. Find your belly button and use your index and middle fingers to measure two finger-widths below it.
2. Imagine placing a marble in the center of your torso at this location.
3. With your next inhale, imagine that you can breathe into the marble, blowing it up like a balloon to about the size of a softball. You should feel expansion in every direction from the starting point to the ending.
4. As you exhale, imagine the softball returning to the size of a marble.

Continue practicing these steps as you employ the following awareness checks.

PELVIC FLOOR—YOUR DOWNSTAIRS

Repeat steps 3 and 4 from the previous exercise while putting your full conscious awareness in your pelvic floor area. This is the area between your legs where your anus and genitals reside. You should feel expansion or pressure down into your pelvic floor when you inhale, and the pressure should subside with each exhale. If you don't feel this at first, don't be frustrated. Most people have a difficult time relaxing the pelvic floor. This is usually the result of years of clenching due to chronic stress and anxiety. We don't often realize just how much tension we hold in this area. Your unconscious-self will tense up muscles to help to protect sensitive areas. Most of us have been in such a chronic state of stress for so long, this area will take some time and conscious effort to relax.

Pelvic Floor Relaxation Technique

One technique to relax the pelvic floor that works for many of my clients is to imagine a four-sided trapezoid using your iliac crests (the part of your pelvis just under your waistline) and your ischia (sometimes called your "sit bones"). Once you have visualized the trapezoid, begin the marble-to-softball breathing exercise, envisioning the trapezoid expanding with every inhale as well. This seems to help people to relax their "downstairs," but don't get frustrated if you need to practice this often to see improvements. Awareness is the foundation of all positive change. Now that you are aware of this tension, you can make positive change by practicing this exercise regularly.

THE SIDES OF THE ABDOMEN

Continue practicing the marble-to-softball exercise, but now, place your hands on the sides of your abdomen. You should feel some expansion here with every inhale, and with each exhale this should subside. This expansion should coincide with the expansion in the pelvic floor, just as if there really is a marble expanding to the size of a softball, displacing matter in your abdomen. For most people, simply putting their conscious awareness here is enough to experience proper expansion, but many people have trouble expanding this area.

One technique to help you improve expansion in this area is to place your hands on your sides to provide some resistance. Simply offering this physical feedback can be enough to make a big change, offering a physical cue for you to breathe into.

THE LOWER BACK

As you practice breathing into the marble, turning it into a softball with every inhale, you should also feel some expansion in your lower back. Place the soft tissue of your thumbs on your lower ribs and use the palms of your hands to feel your lower back. Can you feel expansion here? While it will not be as pronounced as what is happening in your tummy, you should still feel some expansion here with every inhale.

One technique to help you improve expansion in this area is to put your conscious awareness in this place so that when you take an inhale, it is as if you are directing the air to the lower back. Breathe into it as if you have moved your tummy into your lower back. Many practitioners find that doing this also allows them to activate their pelvic floor and sides evenly as well.

THE LOWER RIBS

Continue this exercise. Does it feel as though there is a sphere applying pressure outwardly in every direction from the location we identified earlier? If so, you should feel some pressure expanding upward, as if it is expanding in the shape of an upside-down bowl (a dome) within the ring of your lower rib cage. Your lower ribs should expand slightly.

For those who cannot feel this expansion, it is usually the result of constant tension in your abdominals that you might not be consciously aware of. This generally goes away with regular practice. As you develop a greater sense of internal awareness, breathing into this area becomes very natural.

THE TUMMY

Most people focus too much on the tummy, which is why we are covering it last. When you inhale, breathing the marble into the softball, you should feel expansion in the tummy. This will be the most pronounced area of expansion. However, this expansion does not have to be extreme. Many breathwork practitioners pride themselves on being "belly breathers," sometimes hyperextending the tummy. This might be because they believe that the more extended the tummy gets, the healthier the breath. Of course, some people are doing this to show off. Yes, you read that right. Anytime humans are involved, we will find the strangest things to brag about.

The best way to properly utilize the tummy in each breath is to focus more on expanding the other areas already discussed. This helps you to avoid overextending this area. However, a very useful exercise to ensure that you are only breathing into the first part of the breath wave is to place one hand on your tummy and one hand on your chest. Focusing on producing spherical expansion from the marble to the softball with each inhale, observe your hands. The hand on the tummy should be the only one moving. The chest should be still when practicing this exercise because we are only activating the lower part of the breath wave.

HOW DOES THE BELLY EXHALE?

The diaphragm is an incredible muscle. It is connected to both sides of your brain, allowing you to breathe functionally, even if you experience brain trauma on one side. However, it only goes one direction. You can only inhale with it. To exhale, we use our abdominal muscles. Go ahead. Forcefully exhale, and feel which muscles made it happen. Most of the time, we don't need to forcefully exhale. However, when we do, it is our abdominal muscles that make this possible.

Final note on the belly: The belly should always be the first part of the breath wave to expand and the last to collapse.

Station 2: The Ribs—Using the Intercostal Muscles

When the demands of cellular respiration exceed what can be facilitated by the lower lobes, the next part of the breath wave is ready to accommodate. Because this should only happen when physical needs make it necessary, when the unconscious-self observes this portion of the breath wave becoming active, it infers that you are becoming more active. This isn't at the level of

active of running from a bear or charging a hill. But it is not the level of loung-
ing in the cave or reading a book either. The tone, when activating the ribs
in your breathing, is somewhere in between relaxed and intense. You might
simply refer to it as "active."

The intercostal muscles are a three-layered muscle group that are the primary muscles involved in inhales and exhales. Any time you move your ribs,
you are using your intercostal muscles. This major area of the breath wave
should activate only after the first major area, the belly, has fully activated.
Expanding the ribs expands the middle regions of the lungs, inviting air into
this general area. As we discussed, this middle area of the lungs facilitates
a gas exchange quite well. While it is not as efficient as the lower lobes, it is
more efficient than the upper regions. When the intercostal muscles expand,
the middle area of your lungs expands, reducing the pressure in this part of
your lungs and inviting air to fill the middle.

One way to ensure that your ribs are expanding is to use your hands to
monitor them as they expand. This offers some gentle resistance for your ribs
to expand into. The exercise titled "The Jolly Green Giant," described later in
this chapter, is one effective exercise in ensuring that your ribs are expanding
before exercise or other activities.

The intercostals are also the principal muscles involved in a forceful
exhale. While most of the time we can simply relax these muscles to exhale, if
we need to forcefully exhale from this part of the breath wave, the intercostal
muscles will also make this happen. Go ahead and try another exhale, putting
your conscious awareness on the feeling of the belly expanding fully, then the
ribs expanding; then exhale forcefully, contracting the intercostals first and
then the abdominals.

Station 3: The Chest

When the need for gas exchange has become so great that it cannot be satisfied by the lower lobes and the middle regions of the lungs, it is time to use
the upper areas of the lungs, even though they are not very effective at facilitating gas exchange. If you think about how the unconscious-you interprets
the use of this portion of your breath wave, you might consider what kinds of
situations it might expect you to be in if you need to breathe so fully. As you

might have guessed, this is the part of your lungs that your unconscious-self expects you to use if you are being chased by a bear or charging a hill. The use of this portion of our lungs corresponds with high intensity, and when we use this portion of our lungs, this is the tone that we are bringing to every breath. Sadly, many people who suffer from dysfunctional breathing patterns breathe in this portion of the breath wave regularly, and this is usually connected to mouth breathing, which we will discuss later.

When we breathe into the chest, we recruit what are referred to as accessory breathing muscles. These muscles' primary function is not breathing, but they can be recruited in times of respiratory distress. They include the scalenes, the sternocleidomastoid, the pectoralis major, and the trapezius. These muscles help to expand the upper areas of the lungs, pulling outward and upward.

People generally overuse this part of the breath wave, but I still see a lot of dysfunction in this part of the breath wave due to the problem of poor posture. People who sit at desk jobs or who are constantly using their phones tend to have upper-crossed syndrome, a condition that is typically the result of chronically inhibited neck flexors, rhomboids, and serrati anterior combined with tight pectorals, upper trapezii, and levatores scapulae. This causes the neck to extend forward and the shoulders to droop and fall forward. When people with upper-crossed syndrome try to use the upper part of the breath wave, they can experience back pain, tension, and headaches while never actually fully expanding the upper area of the lungs. In fact, research has shown a nearly 20 percent reduction in lung capacity in people who suffer from upper-crossed syndrome.[2] If you have upper-crossed syndrome, find a personal trainer or a physical therapist for advice. However, for most people, simply looking up, sticking out your chest, and pulling your shoulders back multiple times throughout the day can undo a lot of what has been done by hunching over a computer keyboard or a smart phone.

Adhering to the Breath Wave

As we have touched on already, the unconscious-you is always paying attention. This includes the way you breathe. The literal action of every breath that you take is being monitored by your unconscious-self. And it assumes that you are using the breath in the same order as when you were a baby.

THE TONE AND INFLECTION CHART

Belly breathing (low and slow) = relaxed, calm, confident

Belly and ribs (still controlled but possibly more active) = active, in control, confident

Anything involving the chest = stressed, high intensity, worried

---

Another very important reason why functional breathing follows the breath wave is because functional breathing is efficient breathing. If each breath maximizes the potential gas exchange, you simply don't need to breathe as quickly. As we discussed earlier when examining the language of breath's Rosetta Stone, the ANS, when our breath quickens, we are speaking stress to our unconscious-self. When we breathe slowly, we are speaking relaxation to our unconscious-self. Simply by breathing into our lower lobes, we reduce our need for fast breathing because our needs are being met with the least amount of airflow as possible. Many people breathe into their chests without activating their belly or ribs, and as a result, they have to breathe more breaths per minute to absorb the same amount of oxygen and release the same amount of carbon dioxide. Without realizing it, they are speaking with a stressed tone with every breath they take.

Making an Agreement to Breathe Functionally

Now that we have learned what the breath wave should be like with regard to functional breathing, go back to your videos and examine your current breath wave. Do your inhales follow the order belly ➜ ribs ➜ chest? Are your exhales relaxing in the order of chest ➜ ribs ➜ belly? This is when honest self-appraisal is key. And if you are confused, it is okay to be honest about that too. Even if you have trouble assessing your breathing on your video, you now know what you should focus on in every breath that follows.

But your breath wave isn't something that your conscious-self alone will need to learn. Your breath is where you and your unconscious-self come together. Both your conscious-self and unconscious-self will need to work together to ensure that your breathing will remain functional both when you are consciously controlling your breath and when you unconsciously control your breathing. This takes time, patience, a good sense of humor, and conscious effort. It's not just your conscious-self that has fallen out of practice of functional breathing, it's also your unconscious-self. You need to work as a team to relearn this skill.

Functional Breathing—Posture Is Crucial

Functional breathing depends on good posture because it is built on the structures that make up one's posture. It's important to acknowledge that not everyone can maintain proper posture for reasons that go beyond the conditions described here. Even for those who can, in the modern world, it is common for people to develop postural issues such as upper-crossed syndrome (generally caused by regular desk work and phone use) and lower-crossed syndrome (most commonly caused by regular extended time sitting in chairs). In these cases, one muscle group is generally lengthened or weakened while the opposing muscle group is shortened or tightened. This is not something to be embarrassed about. It is part of the modern human condition. However, these conditions obscure the expression of the breath wave, making it difficult to breathe naturally. The good news is that these conditions are nearly always correctible. It is not within the scope of this book to cover all the corrective measures that one could take to ameliorate these issues, but a simple strategy is to take time each day to flex the muscles that are normally relaxed in these positions and stretch the muscles that are normally tightened. Working with a bodyworker, personal trainer, or physical therapist is also very worthwhile. These conditions either get better or worse. Nothing stays static in the human organism.

Strengthening Breath Wave Muscles

Strengthening our breathing muscles makes every breath more effective. The following are some exercises to use to improve your conscious awareness of your breathing muscles while improving their ability to fire with ease and precision.

Straw Breathing

This is one of the only techniques that allows for breathing in through the mouth. In fact, it uses the resistance of pursed lips to create a training stimulus to help bring awareness to the muscles of the breath wave while strengthening them with repetition. Avoid using this technique more than what is in the following instructions to avoid unnecessary soreness in the diaphragm.

Instructions for Straw Breathing

1. Exhale 70 to 90 percent of the air in your lungs.
2. Purse your lips as if you were drinking out of a straw.
3. Inhale through your pursed lips, using the complete breath wave. You should feel resistance the entire breath, which should provide a challenge to your breathing muscles.
4. Exhale by simply relaxing your breathing muscles, allowing your chest to relax first, then your ribs, then your belly.
5. Repeat thirty times.

For best results, you can practice two sets of thirty breaths per day. However, on your first day or two, just do one set to gauge the fitness of your inspiratory muscles. If you feel sore after only doing one set, you can throttle back your reps until you have conditioned your muscles enough to do one set per day. Then work your way up to two sets, using your awareness to guide you.

Ocean Breathing—Ujjayi Breath

This technique requires some tension in the back of your throat, much like when you fog up a mirror. This tension will provide some resistance to help bring awareness to every tiny station of the breath wave to fully internalize the subtleties of your breath. This should be a gentle tension, and at no time should it be uncomfortable. While this can strengthen your breathing muscles, the primary goal is to use this technique to allow you to become aware of the subtlety of each breath, becoming intimately aware of every microscopic change within the breath wave as you breathe slowly.

Instructions for Ocean Breathing

1. Take a deep breath using the full breath wave.

2. Tense the back of your throat and exhale with your mouth closed, allowing the tension in the back of your throat to slow down the exhale. You should have to use your abdominal muscles to push the breath out as you slowly empty your lungs 90 to 100 percent of the way empty.

3. Then inhale through your nose, using the same gentle tension in the back of your throat, slowly activating the muscles of the breath wave, feeling every subtle change as you slowly flex these muscles.

4. Repeat this process as long as you like, maintaining the gentle tension in your throat to provide each inhale and exhale with resistance.

The Jolly Green Giant

The Jolly Green Giant is a technique used to warm up the breath wave before physical exercise. In a study led by Mitch Lomax, athletes were simply asked to warm up their breathing muscles in the correct breathing pattern before exertion, which led to a 15 percent improvement in performance over the control group.[3] This technique helps our unconscious-self to remember the order in which we want our muscles to fire so that we can focus our conscious attention on our athletic endeavors, and it is based on the way the Jolly Green Giant stands, with his hands on his sides.

Instructions for the Jolly Green Giant Technique

1. In a standing position, place your hands on the sides of your rib cage. This will allow you to provide some gentle resistance while monitoring your intercostal activation.

2. Inhale through your nose, filling the entire breath wave slowly and purposefully, ensuring that you are pulling your breath down in your belly, then expanding your ribs, then your chest.

3. Exhale actively, using your abdominal muscles and collapsing your ribs.

4. Repeat this for ten breaths.

5. Next, speed this up to your "nasal maximum" or as fast as you can inhale and exhale through your nose. Breathe at this pace for a minute.

6. Now speed your breathing up as fast as you can go, allowing yourself to breathe through your mouth if you need to. Repeat this for thirty seconds.

When you are done, you can go to your sport or exercise program with the confidence of knowing that you have warmed up your breathing muscles and are ready for your best performance.

Language Lab 5

We have come to an important place in learning the language of breath! Thus far we have established some important concepts and learned some important exercises. First, we learned about the skill of interoception: we learned to become more consciously aware of the messages we receive from our internal state, which we often overlook or are unaware of. We have learned to use our autonomic nervous system as the Rosetta Stone for our communications between our conscious- and unconscious-selves. We learned to use our heart rate as a cipher to determine our autonomic state, which allows us to decipher what kind of situation our unconscious-self believes we are in or are about to be in. It also allows us to infer whether or not our messages have been received clearly. We have attempted one "phrase" in the form of a breathing technique: "Let's calm down." We learned this technique before we learned how to use the breath wave to add tone and presence to our message.

You might have already attempted to use what you have learned in this section on the breath wave to add a relaxed tone to your message "Let's calm down." That is great! In the next chapter we will combine what we have learned and begin to form the foundations of our long-term practice using the Language of Breath Philosophy. But before we learn more, take some time to do this chapter's language lab. Everything after this point is built on what we have learned.

> Practice the Interoception Exercise at least once per day, being mindful of your breath wave as you practice.

> Practice using your heart rate as a cipher in the way discussed in chapter 5 and notice how improving your breath mechanics speaks a presence of calm into your philia.

> Practice checking in with your breathing periodically. Simply becoming aware of your breath mechanics throughout the day can give you opportunities to retrain this foundational element of breathing and communication within your philia. Remember that breathing should be low in the breath wave, and every breath should be calm, not erratic or in the chest.

> Do whatever you can to improve your posture or at least avoid doing things that will make your posture worse. Your breathing muscles depend on proper placement of your skeleton to ensure that breathing muscles can operate as they should. See a personal trainer or a physical therapist if you need help improving your posture.

8

Active Listening

Let's combine what we have learned and create an even more robust awareness within your philia. Awareness is the foundation of all positive change, which is why the foundation of your practice will be the Awareness Exercise.

The Awareness Exercise combines what we have learned about the autonomic nervous system (the Rosetta Stone), what we learned about interoception (the Interoception Exercise), and what we have learned about functional breathing into one exercise that, when practiced daily, will serve as your new foundational exercise. We are learning to "hear" the unconscious-self as clearly as possible now so that when we learn to speak phrases with techniques later, we will be able to hear its responses.

Do this every day! It can be practiced anywhere and anytime; however, at first, try to practice and learn it in a seated or lying-down position away from distractions.

>>>>>THE AWARENESS EXERCISE

Step 1. Come into a seated or lying-down position. Close your eyes and focus your conscious awareness on ensuring that you have good posture. We might call this a "neutral" spine. Nothing is hyperextended, nothing is slouched. Begin breathing slowly and fully.

Step 2. Inhale, focusing on utilizing the entire breath wave, expanding the belly completely before expanding the ribs, and only when the ribs are fully expanded, expand the chest. As you inhale, become aware of every part of this movement, every microscopic change that occurs, every slight variation of the contraction of each muscle and the expansion that accompanies it. If you can, use your awareness to trace the air as it enters your nostrils and makes its way to your lungs. Observe the qualities of the air, the coolness, the dryness, humidity, and so on. Observe everything: every subtle change that you feel within you.

Step 3. Exhale slowly, relaxing your chest, then your ribs, and only when the ribs are relaxed, relax your belly. As you exhale, become aware of every part of this movement, every micro-scopic change that occurs, every slight variation in each muscle as it relaxes in the proper order, allowing for the release of air. You don't need to push out any air. Just focus on relaxing your breathing muscles in order and allow the natural recoil of your lungs to do the rest. If you can, use your awareness to trace the air as you exhale it through your nostrils. Trace the breath as it leaves your lungs and exits through your nostrils, becoming aware of its properties. Is it warmer, more humid? At the end of your exhale, you should still have some residual air remaining. We call this end point a "neutral lung." We are not emptying the lungs. Again, observe everything as you exhale; every subtle change in the way you feel, no matter how small.

Step 4. Continue to breathe slow full breaths, placing your con-scious attention on your breath wave as you inhale and exhale. Be sure that you have established a clear focus on your breath before going to the next step. Take as long as you need. Do not rush.

Step 5. Now, add a pause at the end of your exhale before begin-ning your next inhale. During this pause, focus on your inner awareness from head to toe. Can you feel your heartbeat in this pause? Where do you feel it? Is it fast? Is it slow? Allow this pause to last as long as is comfortable for you, using the time between breaths to become aware of your internal state.

Repeat this process for at least five minutes, but there is no limit to how long you can practice this exercise.

The Awareness Exercise in Brief

> Inhale, focusing on every part of the inhale.

> Exhale, focusing on every part of the exhale.

> Pause with a neutral lung, focusing on internal awareness.

> Repeat for at least five minutes or longer.

The Awareness Exercise is an effective way to develop internal awareness while retraining both the conscious- and unconscious-self to breathe functionally. The more you practice it, the better. You'll improve your sense of internal awareness, and you'll improve your breath mechanics. The more you practice it, the more you will notice that your breathing is functional in everyday life. Even if it once felt awkward, in time you'll notice that using the breath wave feels natural and normal.

The Awareness Exercise might seem boring for some. If you are one of those people, it means that you should probably practice it even more. As you will see, developing the sense of inner awareness, the sense of interoception, is just as important as learning conscious breathing techniques. Without cultivating awareness, we are just speaking into the dark, unaware of whether we are being heard and unable to hear a response, even if we are.

Some clients ask, what if my mind starts to wander off and I lose focus? The answer is to simply return your focus back to the exercise as soon as you become aware of it. At first, you might drift off into thought quite often, but as you practice, you'll become aware of your conscious-self drifting quite quickly. In time, you'll be able to catch yourself before you actually begin to drift. You will literally become so aware that you can sense your thoughts drift before they do. This is all part of the practice, and it is how we learn to cultivate a strong sense of internal awareness (interoception).

As you continue to practice, you can move on to the Advanced Awareness Exercise. Avoid moving to the Advanced Awareness Exercise before you can regularly avoid drifting off into distracted thoughts. The Advanced Awareness Exercise will ask for even more conscious focus, so be honest with yourself before progressing. Moving too fast too soon will only create more disconnection. That will be harder to undo than just being patient and progressing when you are ready.

The Advanced Awareness Exercise

In the Advanced Awareness Exercise, we can begin to add the element of conscious thinking to the Awareness Exercise. We can observe the effect that our conscious thoughts have on our philia and become aware of how our unconscious-self interprets them. This will vary from person to person, philia to philia. How does your unconscious-self respond to specific thoughts? When you think of something worrisome, does your heart rate increase quickly? Does it increase slowly? Maybe it doesn't increase? Thinking back to what we know about the Rosetta Stone, we begin to learn about the sensitivity of our unconscious-self and how it interprets our conscious thoughts.

Why do we do this? This is valuable information. We want to learn as much as we can about ourselves so we can learn to work in concert. Many of us don't realize how much our thoughts affect our physiological state. This varies wildly from person to person, so it is important to do the work to find out about yourself. You might be someone who has a proclivity for rumination, like me. Or you might be one of the lucky ones who can think about potential problems with very little effect. Adding thoughts to your Awareness Exercise will help you discover your individualized response. You might think you already know, but it will do you good to do the work and really find out.   <<<<<

Before You Begin

To add thoughts to your Awareness Exercise, you need to come into the exercise with a plan. You should try to avoid only thinking one category of thoughts. For instance, don't just think of five different things you are worried about. You might want to begin with something you are grateful for, then move to something that you are worried about, then move to something you are excited about, then move to something that makes you feel angry, then think about someone you care about. The idea is to avoid thinking only negative or positive things. Try to explore the wide range of emotions that you have and think thoughts that evoke them.

Again, if you "mess up" during this exercise, you should just keep going. Continuing might present an opportunity to observe how your unconscious-self reacts to you consciously thinking that you messed up. It's all good. We all mess up now and then anyway.

You can take a short moment to pause between thoughts. We might think of this as "cleansing the palate." If you need a moment to refocus, take it. If you are not reaching for your phone or some other distraction, you're doing just fine.

Practicing the Advanced Awareness Exercise

Begin the Awareness Exercise as usual, becoming fully aware. Try to do this without adding thoughts for at least the first two minutes. The goal is to become very aware of your current state so you can use this as a baseline for the changes you may experience when you add your conscious thoughts.

After you have become fully aware of your state, begin adding thoughts, still focusing on every detail of the inhale, every detail of the exhale, and every subtle feeling within your philia between each breath.

Focus on one thought at a time, using your sense of interoception to become aware of how this thought affects you. You are observing your unconscious-self's reaction to the thought. It might be subtle; it might be overt. Don't judge it good or bad. Just be aware. Do you feel sensations in your chest, in your abdomen, in your back, or elsewhere? Do you feel a change of temperature? How does this thought affect your heart rate? This is all valuable data that we will try to decipher after the exercise.

Move from one thought to the next at will, but don't rush. Sometimes it takes a little while to pick up on the subtle cues that your unconscious-self will send you. Sometimes your unconscious-self will want you to ruminate on a thought, encouraging you to stay fixated on it longer than you initially intended. Take note of this as well. This is all valuable data. But do your best to keep the time spent on each thought as balanced as possible.

After you complete your list of thoughts, spend a few minutes trying to refocus your attention on the original Awareness Exercise, free of added thoughts, bringing your awareness back to your philia every time you are about to get distracted. Try to maintain the original Awareness Exercise at least two minutes before coming out of this practice.

As soon as you come out of the practice, think about how your unconscious-self responded to each thought. For many people, it is helpful to write this down. However, the most important thing is to think about your experience. How did each thought change the way you felt in the exercise? Where did you notice sensations? How quickly did you notice these sensations? Did they make you want to think about the topic more deeply? All of these things tell you more about yourself.

As for me, I tend to feel an emotional response quickly after I think a thought. My heart rate tends to spike when it is about worrisome things or things that make me excited for the future. I tend to feel the urge to think about worrisome things for longer and more deeply than other topics, and I notice the greatest uptick in my heart rate when thinking about worrisome topics as well. I notice that I may feel a sensation in my philia in different places when I think these thoughts, but I tend to feel heavy in my belly when thinking about worrisome things and warm in my chest when thinking about people I love. I could go on and on because I have done this exercise thousands of times, but this is the kind of self-reporting you should expect to do, and in time, you'll see patterns emerge, giving you a better picture of your unconscious-self's patterns.

This is a long-term practice that will help you to know your philia more deeply. However, with regular practice you will quickly be able to determine just how sensitive your unconscious-self is toward thinking certain things. We often go through our days unaware that our thoughts affect our state. Our state also affects our thoughts, and these things affect our actions. So, one of the things I had to learn was that, because my unconscious-self was very sensitive to worrisome thoughts and would quickly activate my sympathetic nervous system, I needed to develop a way of calming my unconscious-self down *before* my state affected my attitudes and outlooks. But because I know that this is a trait of my own personal unconscious-self and I have developed a very high level of internal awareness, I can take actions using the language of breath long before I suffer from what happens if I let this get out of control. My unconscious-self is only trying to keep me safe and help me reach my goals; but in this case, it needs some feedback to have a more appropriate response.

How many times have we "ripped someone's head off" when we weren't really mad at them? It is very common to lash out or make poor judgment calls when our unconscious-self is sounding the alarm bells. While we might use the term "rip someone's head off" as an expression of speech, if our unconscious-self feels threatened enough, it will put us in a state to actually do just that, even if, consciously, when you really think about it, Connie at the office didn't mean anything by her comment that your hair looks "different today."

The Awareness Exercise is our first and most foundational exercise for learning about our philia, helping us to develop a sense of self-awareness that we will learn to rely on as we become better acquainted with ourselves. We might even be able to change the degree to which our unconscious-self reacts to some things with enough practice. However, learning self-awareness within your philia is much like learning about your partner enough to know what will set them off or make them especially happy. The more aware we are, the better partner we can be and the better our team will operate.

Awareness is the foundation of all positive change, and when we increase this awareness, we are ready to build a vocabulary using breathing techniques. We do this not because the techniques are codes to make our machine do what we want, but because we can use this new vocabulary to begin to take an active role in the communications within our philia.

The goal: The primary goal of practicing the Awareness Exercise is to develop your sense of internal awareness so that you will carry this skill into your everyday life. The more we are aware of how we feel, the better we will be able to communicate effectively with our unconscious-self.

Language Lab 6

Now that we have learned the Awareness Exercise, we will fold everything in together!

> Practice the Awareness Exercise every day for at least five to ten minutes. When you are consistently able to maintain your focus without getting distracted, you can move forward to the Advanced Awareness Exercise, but not before this. Just as with learning any language, you won't do yourself any favors by moving faster than your own pace. Your unconscious-self will always have a lot to say; you are learning to become aware of its messages slowly so that you can eventually have the fullest awareness possible.

> Continue to check in with your breath mechanics throughout your day. Remember that calm, functional breathing creates a presence within your philia of balance and calm. As you check in with your breathing, ask yourself, Am I creating the appropriate presence within my philia? Am I taking breaths in a way that adds a tone of calm or tension? How we take each breath conveys the tone and presence that our unconscious-self will notice and respond to. Remember this when checking your breath throughout the day.

> Don't forget to be mindful of your posture. Stand up straight! Stop slouching and look up as often as possible.

9

Building a Vocabulary for Every Occasion

Imagine that you enter a parlor. You come late. When you arrive, others have long preceded you, and they are engaged in a heated discussion, a discussion too heated for them to pause and tell you exactly what it is about. In fact, the discussion had already begun long before any of them got there, so that no one present is qualified to retrace for you all the steps that had gone before. You listen for a while, until you decide that you have caught the tenor of the argument; then you put in your oar.

—KENNETH BURKE, *THE PHILOSOPHY OF LITERARY FORM*

The Unending Conversation

In this chapter we will begin to take an active role in the conversation that is within us, using the phrases that breathing techniques provide to structure our messages. The way you breathe (functional breathing, smoothness, consistency) determines your tone and presence of voice; now you will learn how to structure phrases.

However, it is important to know that, while you might be entering into this conversation consciously for the first time, this is a conversation that has been going on for your whole life, and you might have even been speaking things into it that you didn't even know you were saying. Whether we know it or not, every breath we take sends a message to our unconscious-self, and over time, this can build toward a positive relationship or a negative one.

The good news is that no matter how bad your inner relationship has become over time, things can be improved, and you have already started to make positive changes by learning to breathe functionally and by cultivating your sense of internal awareness. Even if you started with a chaotic relationship, you could build a peaceful one that is strong enough for whatever life throws at you. This will take time and effort, but it is worth the work. You are worth the work.

What Will We Talk About?

If you are worried that you will run out of things to talk about, don't be. The unconscious-you has one primary interest, and that is surviving and thriving. You won't be using breathwork to discuss your unconscious-self's opinion on politics or art—or will you? Let's remember that it will always have an opinion on whatever you are engaging in. (And let's take this moment to remind ourselves that the unconscious-you is just as much you as the conscious-you.) When you watch the news, you might notice that your unconscious-self has something to say. When you view beautiful art, you might notice that your unconscious speaks as well. "This is a potential threat" or "This is something to strive for" are the two most common things we will "hear" our unconscious-selves speak to us. And while it is important to listen to what the unconscious-you has to say, there are times when you need to use your conscious ability to think critically to determine if the unconscious-you needs some words of correction.

For instance, there will be times when you hear some news that makes you worry more than you should. You notice that your autonomic nervous system is activated, and this is interfering with the goals or challenges that you are currently facing. For instance, maybe you are trying to get some sleep, but for some reason, you are worried about something you heard about on the news that morning. The unconscious-you is asking you to use your conscious skill of critical thinking to solve the problem that it believes may lead to a potential danger. However, after thinking critically about the issue, you know that there is no reason to worry about it, or at least there is nothing you can do about it between now and the time you wake up in the morning. This is an important time to speak the language of breath by practicing breathing techniques to speak calm to your unconscious-self.

Being an Attentive Partner

It is important to practice the Awareness Exercise regularly to develop a sense of rapport with your unconscious-self. Using the valuable skill of interoception, the sense of your internal state, you will be listening to the subtle cues from your unconscious-self throughout your day.

Just as with any partnership, effective communication depends on knowing where you stand at any given moment and not ignoring your partner when your partner speaks. While you certainly will use breathing techniques in times of high stress and overwhelm, much of the time you can avoid the buildup of stress over the day if you are aware of it early enough to take proactive steps to communicate calm to your unconscious-self.

If, after practicing the Awareness Exercise, you discover that you easily become stressed when thinking about things that are worrisome, you should add extra time to speak calm into your philia throughout the days when you are worried. A good partner is mindful of the other; listen to your partner and communicate early and often. Don't wait for your unconscious-self to have to scream!

Knowing Your Role

Your unconscious-self is incredibly smart and can process vast amounts of information quickly to make sense of the world and adjust your physiological expression to match the situation. When your unconscious-self responds and reacts, even when it jumps to the wrong conclusions, it is doing its job. It is using a time-tested survival strategy that kept your ancestors alive and allowed for you to be here today. But your conscious interpretation plays an important role as well. The feeling of being excited and the feeling of being worried often depend on your conscious interpretation of the situation. It is up to your conscious-self to do its part by using your conscious ability to think critically about the situation to inform your unconscious-self if corrections need to be made to your team's reaction.

Our unconscious-self only lives in the present, but your conscious-self can think in the present, the past, and the future. This gives you the opportunity to think about future events to prepare your philia for future situations, putting your philia in the best possible state to meet whatever challenges that situation holds. Because you consciously know about future situations, you can take the lead and prepare your philia to be in the best possible state to enter them when the time comes.

The primary role that you are responsible for, as the conscious side of your philia, is interpreting the true nature of the situation so that your philia can work as a well-informed team. Using the phrases we will learn in this chapter, we can assist our unconscious-self in managing your unified state. The healthiest version of yourself is a team, and everyone on a team has a role to play. Your unconscious-self is doing its job. Now that we have discussed our roles, let's learn methods of communicating within your team.

Breathing Notation

Most breathing techniques involve developing a cadence of breath. This is done by measuring the four corners of the breath, which are the inhale, a full-lungs apnea, the exhale, and a neutral-lungs apnea. While most breathing techniques have names, many are simply known by the ratios between these four variables.

For instance, one of the techniques we will use is commonly known as Box Breathing. It gets this name because it uses a balanced inhale, full-lungs apnea, exhale, and neutral-lungs apnea. The four equal sides of the breath are like the four equal sides of a box, making Box Breathing a descriptive name for this breathing technique.

When writing breathing notation, we always use the following order:

inhale ➡ full-lungs apnea ➡ exhale ➡ neutral-lungs apnea

So, using breathwork notation, Box Breathing would be written: 4,4,4,4. This denotes a breath that is inhaled for four counts, held with a full lung for four counts, exhaled for four counts, and held with a neutral lung for four counts. Typically, each count is measured in seconds, but the ratio takes priority. Therefore, if you are counting off for Box Breathing and your four count is a little more or less than exactly four seconds, don't worry. Having said this, a clock or a metronome is the ideal tool for helping you to count time. Avoid using things that might speed up or slow down, like your heartbeats.

Defining Apneas

An apnea is a breath hold. This can be done with any degree of fullness or emptiness. Unless otherwise specified, however, when using breathwork notation, it is assumed that the first apnea is full, and the second apnea is neutral.

Full-Lungs Apnea: A full-lungs apnea is fairly self-explanatory; however, many practitioners are unsure of just how full the lungs need to be in order to qualify as "full." Suffice to say that if you feel full, you have successfully completed a full-lungs apnea. Yes, there are some "fulls" that are fuller than others. As we go forward, assume that you don't need to have such a fullness that there is a positive pressure coming from within your lungs unless specified. Just fill your lungs to a comfortable fullness and hold without bearing down or squeezing.

Neutral-Lungs Apnea: In a neutral-lungs apnea, you are completely relaxed. To get to a neutral-lungs apnea, just allow your lungs to naturally recoil. We don't push. We don't use any muscles at all. There will be some residual air left over after the lungs recoil, and this is the neutral lung. When we hold our breath with a neutral apnea, we simply relax our breathing muscles and cease breathing.

Empty-Lungs Apnea: It is rare that we will ever use an empty-lungs apnea. To achieve an empty-lungs apnea, you use your abdominals and intercostal muscles to empty your lungs completely and close your glottis to ensure that the negative pressure in your lungs does not invite a new breath in.

Where Most People Get Techniques Wrong

When people find out that I am a breathworker, it is common for them to ask me questions like "What is a breathing technique that will help me . . ." and then say a specific thing like ". . . go to sleep on Sunday nights?" ". . . be more confident on dates?" ". . . lose weight?" It is also common to be asked for things such as "What's a technique for controlling allergies? COPD? arachnophobia?" Of course, they are stuck in the old mind-body paradigm that frames everything as a code to input into our machine for an output. While we can use breathwork to work on illness and irrational fears such as the ones I mentioned, we have to change our paradigm if we are going to make meaningful progress. Assuming you didn't skip over my previous discussion on this point, you should understand this.

However, paradigms are difficult to break, and even the most dedicated practitioner needs reminders. Here is your reminder. You are not a robot; you are a relationship. The techniques we will learn in this chapter are foundational phrases in the Language of Breath Philosophy for the purpose of working with yourself instead of against it. They are not codes or tricks or commands.

Even a perfectly executed technique will only be effective if you take into consideration that your unconscious-self also has goals and concerns. You are a philia, a relationship. Breathwork is not barking orders. It is learning to create a positive relationship that will ultimately lead to cooperation toward a common goal. We want the same thing: to survive and thrive in this world. So, while we learn to speak, never forget that the voice of your conscious-self is not the only one that counts, and you will need to be attentive if you want to make this relationship work.

Two Things to Think about Before Practicing Techniques

Hello? Did You Get That?

When practicing most breathing techniques, you should expect to repeat the technique for at least two minutes before your unconscious-self will begin to respond. While this time will vary from person to person and from situation to situation, expect to spend between two to five minutes practicing a technique before you begin to feel the unconscious-self reply.

Practice the Art of Conversation

If you want to get the most out of learning breathwork as a language, I recommend practicing the Awareness Exercise for a few minutes before and after each of the following techniques as you begin training. Consider this the equivalent of practicing any other language. Time spent practicing interaction in a controlled environment will give you more confidence to speak up in real-life situations.

Practicing Techniques

The following are techniques, or phrases, that can be used to communicate with your unconscious-self. Remember, these are not codes or commands. We are speaking to a part of ourselves that is simply trying to put us in the best state to take actions based on the information it has available. Approach your communication with love and a sense of humor, remembering that with practice, your ability to communicate will improve.

Ratio Breathing

Ratio Breathing refers to breathing cadences that use a consistent ratio between inhales and exhales and do not include apneas. Ratio Breathing can be used to send a message of excitement or relaxation to the unconscious-self using the vagus nerve. While there are many combinations you can use, we will focus on the two primary ratios.

1:2 RATIO—"LET'S CALM DOWN"

This is an easy-to-use technique where every exhale will equal twice the length of the inhale. This stimulates the vagus nerve, which sends a strong message to the unconscious-self to relax. This technique is scalable, which means that you can begin with a ratio that is comfortable, and as you become more relaxed, you can encourage this relaxation by lengthening each breath by the same ratio.

For instance, you might only be comfortable with 2,0,4,0 at first (inhale for 2 seconds, no full-lungs apnea, an exhale for four seconds, and no neutral-lungs apnea), but after two or three minutes, you find that you can tolerate a pace of 3,0,6,0. Perhaps you can relax even more and after two or three minutes of practice, you can extend your breaths even further to 4,0,8,0.

"Let's calm down from this excited state!"	2,0,4,0
"Now that we are a little less excited, let's calm down a little more."	3,0,6,0
"It's safe enough to go to sleep if we want to."	4,0,8,0

If you are trying to calm down, begin with the slowest cadence that you can comfortably perform, and then work your way slower until you are where you want to be. While a cadence of 2,0,4,0 can help bring the philia out of hyper-excitement, if you are already relaxed, this cadence will likely speak more excitement into your philia. Remember that awareness is the foundation of the positive change that you want to make.

A WORD ON TONE AND PRESENCE

When trying to calm down, try to use as little of the breath wave as possible. If you must use a full breath, that is not necessarily a bad thing, but with each breath, focus on relaxing more and more until you only need the belly part of the breath wave.

THE SOLDIER'S TECHNIQUE—"LET'S CALM DOWN"

When I train first responders, military, athletes, fighters, and other people who regularly engage in intense physical and mental challenges, they cannot always afford to use any of their conscious processing power to focus on counting off times. This is when I teach them the Soldier's Technique, which is simplified 1:2 Ratio Breathing without any counting. This is also the first thing that I ask people who are suffering from panic attacks or phobias to do when they are experiencing symptoms. To perform the Soldier's Technique, simply extend your exhale as long as you can comfortably extend it. Inhale as quickly as you need, but put your focus on keeping your exhale as smooth and lengthy as you can without causing yourself to feel breathlessness. This gives you most of the benefits of the 1:2 ratio technique but can be done when you are in intense situations or when you can't focus enough to keep time.

An Example Calm-Down Sequence

The Soldier's Technique ➜ 2,0,4,0 ➜ 3,0,6,0 ➜ 4,0,8,0

HUMMING—"LET'S CALM DOWN"

Humming is a way to comfortably lengthen the exhale. Many find it to be easier than the Soldier's Technique. Simply inhale to full lungs and hum as you exhale as long as you can. Repeat as many times as you need. Humming has also been shown to increase production of nitric oxide, which naturally relaxes blood vessels, opening them for improved blood flow.[1]

2:1 RATIO BREATHING—"LET'S GET EXCITED!"

The 1:2 ratio can be reversed to 2:1 to encourage excitement. When practicing this technique, practitioners generally stick to short bursts of two minutes to ensure that they do not become overexcited. While pumping up some energy is great, too much activation can be stressful. So, as you practice these techniques, use your awareness and take breaks to reassess before repeating.

When we inhale, we inhibit vagal stimulation. Lengthening the inhale and minimizing the exhale provides a gentle message that now is an appropriate time to add a little more energy and alertness. The most common cadence is 4,0,2,0, but this cadence can be lengthened or shortened depending on just how excited you would like to encourage your unconscious-self to be. The way to determine what works best for you is to experiment.

A WORD ON TONE AND PRESENCE

When the goal is to get excited, the ribs and chest should be active. I hesitate to tell clients that when activation is their goal, they can just use the top of their breath wave, because I try to discourage anything that could lead to dysfunctional breathing habits later on. However, if your goal is to increase your energy, practicing the 2:1 ratio using only the top of the breath wave (ribs and chest or just the chest) is an effective way to do this without getting dizzy or light-headed. When you do this, you might notice how similar it feels to gasping. This is not by mistake. The gasp is a natural autonomic response to a sudden stressor. An interesting thing about the gasp is that if it is done on purpose, it tends to send a stressed response to the unconscious-self. This can be beneficial when you are tired and need some energy, but it should be avoided in long sessions to avoid putting yourself into an unwanted state of anxiety.

Balanced Breathing

Balanced Breathing gets its name from a breathing cadence with a one-to-one balance between inhales and exhales. Any breathing that has equal time for inhale as exhale without any apneas is a form of Balanced Breathing. For instance, 6,0,6,0 is a breathing cadence that has a six-second inhale and a six-second exhale without any apneas between. This is just one way to breathe with balance.

Balanced Breathing is a way to send a message to your unconscious-self to be calm and ready to adapt. Even when it is fast, its regularity adds assurance to your unconscious-self, unlike the erratic breathing patterns that are common when in a stressed or panicked state. In fact, I advise the use of Balanced Breathing to anyone who is wondering which breathing technique to start with or to master first. Simply learning to master a technique using your breathing muscles in a balanced and consistent way is a major accomplishment and can become a baseline for building a positive rapport with your unconscious-self.

The slower your breathing, the more relaxing your message will be for your unconscious-self; the faster, the more energizing. However, there is a sweet spot that your unconscious-self will interpret as a call to stimulate the baroreceptors in your large blood vessels to lower blood pressure, improve heart rate variability, and elevate mood. This is commonly referred to as Resonance Frequency Breathing, a name coined by biofeedback scientist Evgeny Vaschillo, who first discovered its benefits on the cardiovascular system.[2]

RESONANCE FREQUENCY BREATHING—SPEECH THERAPY

Resonance Frequency Breathing could be described as speech therapy within the framework of the Language of Breath Philosophy. This is primarily because it is not just a kind of breathwork that we do simply to speak a message in the moment; it has cumulative effects that can benefit the overall health of our philia.

Simply put, to practice Resonance Frequency Breathing, you breathe at a balanced cadence at a speed of approximately six breaths per minute. Since the average person breathes approximately twelve to twenty breaths per minute, this is significantly slower than everyday breathing. Each breath should be soft, light, and quiet.

Your heart is connected to every breath you take. It speeds up as you breathe in, and it slows down as you breathe out. Practicing Resonance Frequency Breathing maximizes this variance, naturally improving your heart rate variability (HRV). HRV is an indicator of the resilience of your heart to deal with stress, reduce blood pressure, and improve overall mood.[3]

The science of Resonance Frequency Breathing is complicated, but research suggests that Balanced Breathing at approximately the pace of 5,0,5,0 stimulates and improves a part of our nervous system referred to as the ventral vagal complex, also known as "the social engagement system"—a collection of pathways that is unique to mammals and allows us to form bonds and connections with other mammals within our group. It also plays a major role in our HRV health. In the modern world, we experience disconnection and chronic unchecked stress, causing these important pathways to weaken. The improvements in HRV show that practicing Balanced Breathing at approximately six breaths per minute for twenty minutes per day will overhaul the health of your ventral vagal complex in less than six weeks of daily practice, which is not only good for your physical health but improves your ability to form new connections with other people.[4]

Instructions for Balanced Breathing (5,0,5,0)

1. For best results, lie down or sit comfortably in a chair so that you can be completely relaxed.

2. With a neutral spine, inhale through your nose for five seconds, using the least amount of the breath wave as is comfortable.

3. Exhale through the nose for five seconds, relaxing the breath.

4. Repeat steps 2 and 3 for at least ten to twenty minutes.

We think of Resonance Frequency Breathing as speech therapy within the framework of learning breath as a language because practicing this very simple breathing cadence on a consistent basis seems to improve the degree to which the unconscious-self responds to all breathing techniques.

Box Breathing—"Let's Stay Focused, Relaxed, and Centered"

As we discussed earlier in the section titled "Breathing Notation," Box Breathing is named after its use of even sides—the four sides of the breath. The most common cadence for Box Breathing is 4,4,4,4.

Instructions for Box Breathing (4,4,4,4)

1. With a neutral spine, inhale through your nose for four seconds, using functional breathing to fill your lungs.

2. Hold your breath with full lungs for four seconds.

3. Exhale through the nose for four seconds, relaxing the chest, then the ribs, and then the belly.

4. Hold your breath with a neutral lung for four seconds.

5. Repeat steps 1 through 4 for at least two minutes.

CHANGING THE BOX SIZES CHANGES THE MESSAGE

Your box can be expanded to add more relaxation or tension to the message. For instance, you might struggle to maintain a box of 7,7,7,7 because you find it difficult to breathe at such a slow cadence. If you stick to this cadence despite the added stress of air hunger, your unconscious-self might respond in a number of ways. Depending on your philia, your unconscious-self might respond by increasing your ability to focus. It might also respond by relaxing. Or it could do something completely different. This is where experimenting is helpful. Your philia is a relationship all your own. When you adjust techniques, always be willing to check in with your unconscious-self to see how it interprets your message.

A WORD ON TONE AND PRESENCE

The Box Breathing Technique is a very versatile tool for messaging your unconscious-self. By keeping all sides of the box even, you are encouraging your unconscious-self to stay balanced and centered. You're saying that it is not a time to freak out and it's not a time to take a nap. This is generally great for improving focus. You can modulate the tone and presence in your message by deciding how much of your breath wave to use. The fuller your breath wave, the more excited your tone.

If you only use the lower end of your breath wave (belly), your message will have a more relaxed tone. Of course, all of this depends on how your unconscious-self is feeling. If your unconscious-self is already excited, it will be difficult to use only your belly. In this case, if you are trying to speak more relaxation into your message, just try to use as little of the breath wave as possible until your unconscious-self becomes a little more relaxed, allowing you to use even less of the breath wave. Be patient with your unconscious-self. Remember that it usually takes about two minutes to begin to respond.

BOX BREATHING—THE GREAT PREGAME PEP TALK

Box Breathing can be practiced for as long as you want to use it. It is a great way to reassure the unconscious-self that everything is okay, but we should still stay awake and alert. Sometimes we might call this a state of "stay and play."

When the conscious-self ruminates or is nervous about a future event, the unconscious-self will try to do what any good partner would do and change the philia's physical expression, increasing stress hormones and activating the sympathetic nervous system to prepare to fight or flee the situation. Of course, this might be exactly what the philia needs, but most of the time, this just leads to expectation anxiety.

Expectation anxiety usually does more harm than good. It robs us of calm while there is no reason to be activated, and it wears us down before the time when we might actually need the extra energy. We also tend to make poorer choices when we experience anxiety. To be best suited to jump into action when needed, the ideal state is centered and balanced. This is the message that Box Breathing sends to the unconscious-self.

BOX BREATHING—REASSURE THE PHILIA THROUGHOUT THE DAY

Box Breathing is the most underrated breathing technique. It sends such a perfect message of centeredness and focus to the unconscious-self that most people should practice it throughout the day once or twice just to bring the team together as a reminder that we can stay calm and alert.

The ANS Activation Technique—"Wake Up!"

The ANS Activation Technique is a way to lovingly shout to your unconscious-self, "Let's get up and go!" It is practiced as follows:

Instructions for the ANS Activation Technique

1. In a seated or standing position, empty your lungs completely.
2. Inhale, using short sniffs through the nose as you fill your breath wave completely.
3. Exhale all the air quickly through your nose.
4. Repeat steps 2 and 3 between three and ten times.
5. Wait a minute before doing another set.
6. Repeat this process as many times as needed.

This technique will look a little like you are fighting a sneeze as you inhale and a little like a controlled sneeze through your nose as you exhale. The more sniffs you can do on the inhale, the better, and if you let a little air out between sniffs, it is okay. This technique utilizes the gasp reflex and is not dependent on the gas exchange. If practiced correctly, you will not feel light-headed. Instead, you will begin to feel energy because you have just sent a loud conscious message to the unconscious to wake up and energize.

Triangles

Triangle techniques include apneas to lengthen each breath and to add meaning to your message. The interesting thing about apneas is that they often send different messages, depending on the person. We will also use triangles in chapter 11 when we learn to train our CO_2 tolerance.

Triangles usually use equal ratios. For example, the most common Top Triangle notation is: 4,4,4,0. This means that the inhale, the full-lungs apnea, and the exhale are all done for the same amount of time. The triangle can expand (for example: 5,5,5,0) or it can contract (3,3,3,0) depending on what kind of message you are intending to send. If you recall what we learned from the Rosetta Stone of the autonomic nervous system, the faster we breathe, the more we speak activation to our unconscious-self. So, the smaller your triangle, the more likely your message will be interpreted as activating. The larger your triangle, the slower you will breathe, which is likely to enhance a message of relaxation.

TOP TRIANGLE—"WE NEED ENERGY!" OR "WE NEED TO RELAX!"

While Top Triangle usually sends a message of activation, about a third of my clients over the years have noticed that this technique sends a message of relaxation. The best way to test to see how your unconscious-self will respond is to use your heart rate as your cipher. If your heart rate increases, your unconscious-self is interpreting this technique as a message to activate. If your heart rate goes down, your unconscious-self is interpreting this technique as a message to relax.

Instructions for Top Triangle (4,4,4,0)

1. Using a neutral spine and a full breath wave, inhale for four seconds.
2. With full lungs, hold your breath for four seconds.
3. Exhale for four seconds to neutral.
4. Repeat steps 1 through 3.

Like most techniques in this section, the majority of people require at least two minutes of this technique before they begin to notice a clear change in the way they feel or in their heart rate. However, many people practice Top Triangle for much longer. It all depends on the beginning state of your philia and the state you would like to achieve.

BOTTOM TRIANGLE—"LET'S SLOW DOWN AND RELAX"

Bottom Triangle uses balanced inhales and exhales with a neutral-lungs apnea between breaths. This is a technique that helps to slow down breathing using a relaxing pause. It can be visualized as an equilateral triangle with equal lengths inhale and exhale as its sides and with a neutral-lungs apnea as its base. This is the technique we use when practicing the Awareness Exercise, so you have already practiced it before. The only difference is that Bottom Triangle should be done at a consistent pace, whereas the Awareness Exercise does not require any specific pace.

Bottom Triangle can be practiced using any time count that you like. However, remember that the faster you breathe, the more your autonomic nervous system will perceive that you want to become more active. Most people begin with a count of 4,0,4,4 and expand their triangle as they become more and more relaxed. As with most techniques, expect to repeat this technique at a single speed for around two minutes before your unconscious-self will respond.

A WORD ON TIME AND TONE

This technique can be practiced for minutes to hours. This technique can be practiced with a full breath wave or a minimal breath wave, depending on your comfort level; however, if you want to use this technique to encourage your unconscious-self to relax and feel safe, you should only use the belly without activating the entire breath wave.

Instructions for Bottom Triangle (4,0,4,4)

1. Using a neutral spine and a minimal breath wave, inhale for four seconds.
2. Exhale for four seconds to a neutral lung.
3. Hold a neutral-lungs apnea for four seconds.
4. Repeat steps 1 through 3.

The Cadence of Bliss—"Let's Feel Good!"

There are plenty of times in life where we need a little feel-good boost. When we use this technique, we are asking our unconscious-self for a little boost of bliss. It can be used any time. Many people use it before they need to make an uncomfortable phone call. Others use it before they speak in public. It can also be used to encourage your unconscious-self to stop worrying at night so you can get some sleep. Simply put, this technique is a pleasure to practice. I like to think of it as inviting my unconscious-self to have a beer; but instead of having the side effects of alcohol, this technique is safe and healthy. I can't promise it won't be habit-forming, but this is a habit that you won't regret.

Instructions for Cadence of Bliss (4,7,8,0)

1. With a neutral spine, inhale through the complete breath wave through your nose, being mindful to expand your ribs as much as possible for four seconds.
2. Hold your breath with full lungs, feeling the pressure within your ribs as you hold for seven seconds. To supercharge the experience, smile during the hold. Trust me.
3. Exhale through your mouth or nose, relaxing your chest, then the ribs, then the belly to a neutral lung. This exhale should be even and smooth, avoiding the tendency to let too much out in the beginning and too little out at the end.
4. Repeat steps 1 to 3 between four and eight times.
5. Return to normal breathing for at least one minute before repeating this sequence. Going longer than eight breaths in this sequence can result in a diminished message that your unconscious-self will not respond to as robustly.

Peaceful Apneas—"Let's Feel Good and Energize"

Peaceful Apneas are much like the Cadence of Bliss, but they are much easier to do quickly and when you don't have the focus to count. However, unlike the Cadence of Bliss, because there is no extended exhale in this technique, it can also give some people an added boost of energy.

Instructions for Peaceful Apneas

1. With a neutral spine, inhale through the complete breath wave through the nose, being mindful to expand the ribs as much as possible.

2. Hold your breath with full lungs, feeling the pressure within your ribs as you hold for two or three seconds. To supercharge the experience, smile during the hold.

3. Exhale through your mouth or nose, relaxing your chest, then the ribs, then the belly to a neutral lung. If exhaling through your mouth, make a swishing sound to slow your exhale and help maintain relaxation.

4. Repeat steps 1 to 3 for three repetitions.

5. Return to normal breathing for at least one minute before repeating this sequence.

Important Notes on Breathing Techniques

Now that we have learned some phrases in the language that our unconscious-self understands, there are some important things to keep in mind.

Are You Forcing a Conversation?

I had a client who just couldn't shake the mind-body machine paradigm. He came to me because he was a CEO who often felt uneasy while flying, something he had to do often for his company. He learned some phrases from this chapter, which he conceptualized as "commands to make the body calm down." He practiced them with me on our calls, but later he admitted he never practiced the Awareness Exercise and only randomly practiced any of the techniques we learned.

Then one day he found himself feeling intense anxiety as the flight attendant on his plane closed the door and prepared for takeoff. It was then that he remembered to use Ratio Breathing, but instead of starting with using his awareness to choose an appropriate cadence, he went straight to 4,0,8,0, which he felt would be the best because, in his mind, it was a command to "go to sleep." What he found was that he had a difficult time performing it comfortably. He strained to force the four counts on the inhale, and he couldn't even get to a five count on the exhale. This caused him to feel even more stressed because now he felt like he was suffocating on top of his fear of flying. At this point, rather than listening to his unconscious-self's concerns and adjusting his cadence to something more comfortable, he continued to force himself to suffer because he looked at the technique as a command for his machine rather than a message within his internal relationship with his unconscious-self, which was very alarmed. After multiple attempts to force the technique, he gave up and had a terrible flight. What happened here?

This is an example of someone neglecting to listen to his unconscious-self and just making things worse. Most of breathwork involves working with levels of autonomic arousal. In other words, much of what your conversations with your unconscious-self will be about is the appropriate level of excitement that your philia should adopt as you adapt to each situation. A practitioner forcing a breathing technique even though it was uncomfortable to do is equivalent to yelling at someone who is having a panic attack to "calm down." You're not matching your message to the level that will speak to your unconscious-self's level of concern. This is why we have many techniques that can be used depending on what is appropriate. Remember that your breath is the action that you share with your unconscious-self. Don't turn it into a tug-of-war.

Start with a technique that is reasonably easy to perform in your current state. As your unconscious-self calms down, we can switch to a technique that will continue to move the conversation in the direction we would like. We never force a technique. Instead, we switch through techniques to find one that can be performed with relative ease.

Guiding the Conversation—Using Techniques in a Sequence

Once you have learned how your unconscious-self responds to each of these techniques, you can begin to experiment with putting them together into a sequence based on where you would like to direct the overall state of your philia. Think of this much like taking an active role in a conversation and guiding it in a direction that you would like it to go. This is what my CEO client should have done, and after his aforementioned experience, what he eventually learned to do.

For instance, you might begin with simply extending your exhale to bring your philia out of a high state of excitement or anxiety. Then, after you become a little more settled, you might switch to Box Breathing to encourage your philia to be balanced and focused. You might stick with that technique for a long time, and then choose another one to guide your team to the best state for your situation. Then, using your developed sense of awareness, you might leave the breathing to your unconscious-self, confident that your regular practice of functional breathing has been internalized to the point that you don't have to constantly be in control of it.

Eventually, this becomes a normal part of your conscious life. You'll Box Breathe on the way to work, using your sense of awareness to put your philia in the best possible state for the challenges of the day. Then you can just let your unconscious-self take over while simply maintaining a level of internal awareness throughout the day.

When your unconscious-self speaks up and says something like "This could potentially be dangerous," you will understand that this excited feeling (increased heart rate, heightened sense of alertness, and so on) is coming from your partner, who is doing its job. Then you can consciously appraise the situation and check in with yourself. Maybe this is a stressful situation in which you will need to think creatively to solve problems. In such an instance, you might become aware that you are too activated to focus. This is an opportunity to lengthen your exhales for a while, meeting your unconscious-self where it is, and throttling down your team's reaction. Maybe you decide to have a little feel-good session by doing the Cadence of Bliss (4,7,8,0) for a few breaths. After that, you might feel so good that you let your unconscious-self take over the breathing for a while until you need to send another message to calm down or perk up. Your unconscious-self is always listening, always trying to put your philia in the best state to meet the situation. Now you are too. This is what a healthy team looks like!

Creating Your Own Phrases

All techniques were created by someone. This is generally a process of experimenting with an idea and using your awareness to know how your message was received. Just as when we are learning any language, we benefit from learning common phrases, such as the ones we learned in this chapter. However, as you become more familiar with yourself and how your philia operates, you might decide to create your own technique. That is great! Here are some quick tips on the "linguistics" of breathing techniques.

INHALES   Lengthened inhales tend to make your message more sympathetic dominant. In other words, they are more likely to send a message of excitement or stress. Lengthen inhales to add activation to your message. Shorten inhales to limit activation in your messages.

EXHALES   Lengthened exhales tend to make your message more parasympathetic dominant. In other words, they are more likely to make your message more relaxing. Lengthen exhales to add relaxation to your messages. Shorten exhales to limit relaxation to your message.

FULL-LUNGS APNEAS   While full-lungs apneas can add excitement to your message, an extended full-lungs apnea with some tension in your ribs can be quite relaxing when you release it. This is the primary reason why the Cadence of Bliss (4,7,8,0) is so relaxing for most people. Short full-lungs apneas help you slow down your breathing, which can lengthen the breathing process, adding relaxation to your overall message. However, for some, they can also be quite activating. The best way to determine if a full-lungs apnea is right for your message is to experiment and to use your awareness to infer how your unconscious-self replies.

NEUTRAL-LUNGS APNEAS   Neutral-lungs apneas are generally quite relaxing unless they are held for long periods of time. We will learn more about the CO_2 fear response in chapter 11, but as long as you avoid holding a neutral-lungs apnea to the point of inducing stress, these are generally great ways to add relaxation to your message.

Remember, the Healthiest You Is a Team

As you practice communicating with yourself using these techniques and the many more you will learn in this book, just remember that the healthiest version of you is one that works as a team. Using your conscious ability to think critically about your situation allows you to work with your unconscious-self, providing valuable information so that it can do its best job for your team.

Language Lab 7

Now we are in a really fun place where you can begin to actively engage with your unconscious-self. It is time to begin to make a positive conscious impact on your philia by sending messages via the techniques we learned in this chapter. Use the Awareness Exercise to help you determine whether your unconscious-self received the message and interpreted it in the way that you meant to send it. Breathwork is all about developing your awareness while speaking with every breath.

> Practice the Awareness Exercise or the Advanced Awareness Exercise every day for at least five to ten minutes. If you have not mastered the Awareness Exercise, don't worry. This is a lifelong practice, and it should not be rushed. Be patient with yourself and enjoy the journey. Feel free to practice this exercise longer than ten minutes per day as well.

> Continue to check in with your breath mechanics throughout your day and be mindful of your posture. Remember that calm, functional breathing creates a presence within your philia of balance and calm.

> Practice all of the techniques described in this chapter, but start a "favorites list" early on that you practice daily. While you can practice all of these techniques daily as you are beginning your practice, it is better to practice three or four often rather than eight or nine just once. However, this is where it is important to develop your own relationship with yourself. Really explore this beautiful partnership within you!

> A fun challenge is to observe your heart rate and try to use one of the techniques in this chapter to speed it up or slow it down, remembering what we learned about the heart rate and its place within the Rosetta Stone of the ANS. As you do this, don't just focus on the numbers, however. Use your sense of interoception as well, forming a complete understanding of how the unconscious-self is interpreting your messages.

10

Love Your Nose

I don't know how you feel about your nose, but I think your nose is amazing. Your nose filters, humidifies, and adjusts the temperature of every breath you take. But so often, we humans opt to breathe through our mouths instead of using the sinuses. Why do we do this?

Most of us are unaware that it matters whether we breathe with our mouth or our nose, so we don't even think about it. The mouth offers less resistance to breathing, so we often just opt for the mouth because it is easier. This is especially true for public speakers or people who talk a lot. But to mouth-breathe is to forfeit a part of your anatomy that was specifically built for breathing and making every breath you take healthier and more effective.

The reality is that mouth breathing is a common cause of breathing dysfunction specifically because it does not offer the resistance that nasal breathing offers. Nasal breathing offers 50 percent more resistance than mouth breathing, which encourages the diaphragm to activate more effectively, increasing the vacuum of the lungs with every inhalation. This results in a 10 to 20 percent increase in oxygen absorption. Nasal exhalation also improves gas transport by increasing the pressure within the lungs during exhalation.[1] Therefore, even when respiratory demands are high, nasal breathing is superior to mouth breathing.

When we inhale through our nose, we are also inhaling nitric oxide, a vasodilation-inducing molecule released in our paranasal sinuses that is carried down into our lungs with each breath, relaxing and opening our airways to keep our alveoli open and healthy.[2] It has a positive effect on smooth muscle tone, circulation within the lungs, and mucus production, the first line of defense against pathogens when they reach the lungs.[3]

However, much of what we inhale through the nose never makes it past our *turbinates*, the three mucus lined shelves within our sinuses that are shaped much like elongated shells, which is why they are also sometimes called "conchas." The turbinates humidify, warm, and filter the air passing through our sinuses, trapping particles in a layer of mucus, and disposing of potential irritants and threats before they can irritate the rest of our respiratory system. When we inhale through our mouth, we inhale harsh raw air directly into our lungs, potentially inviting irritation, inflammation, and infection with every breath.

Perhaps one of the most common breathing dysfunctions is chest breathing, the tendency to use only the top of the breath wave while breathing, excluding the two areas of the lungs that facilitate the most effective gas exchange and signaling to your unconscious-self that you are in a potentially dangerous situation. Since the upper third of the lungs is the least effective at absorbing oxygen, chest breathing requires more breaths per minute to achieve the same gas exchange as would be needed with functional breathing. When we breathe fast, especially when activating the part of our breath wave that is normally associated with full breaths that we might take when running from a predator, this activates the autonomic nervous system to become sympathetic dominant. The unconscious-you prepares for a potential threat, even though all you might be doing is sitting at your desk. When we mouth-breathe, we also release excess amounts of CO_2, which can lead to a reduced CO_2 tolerance. This is explained in greater depth in chapter 11, on CO_2 training, but the result is a heightened sensitivity to CO_2 that tends to cause fast and erratic breathing patterns, which again send signals of distress and potential danger to our unconscious-self.

Many breathwork styles use mouth breathing, while others use nasal inhalations while exhaling through the mouth. While the latter is better than plain mouth breathing, the ideal way to breathe in any circumstance is purely nasal. While this might be challenging, maybe even painful at first, in this section we will learn strategies to get you to 100 percent nasal breathing, even when you are playing sports or doing intense heavy breathing. Research shows that when we exhale through the mouth we are exhaling 42 percent more water than if we exhale though the nose.[4] This is especially impactful for athletes, but it also affects anyone who is interested in deep breathwork—the kinds we will get into later in this book as well as other popular styles today. The exhale helps to keep the sinuses warm, moist, and malleable, so while using nasal inhales with mouth exhales is better than mouth breathing alone, it has actually been shown to cause nasal obstruction, reducing one's nasal capacity.[5]

From this point on, make a promise to yourself to do your very best to breathe in and out of your nose only. While this might be difficult to do at first, it gets easier over time. Before long, you'll be the weird cousin at the family get-together who shows off just how fully and quickly you can breathe through your nose. But, until then, let's discuss some strategies that work well for most people.

When Exercising

The most effective way to increase your nasal breathing capacity is to engage in 100 percent nasal breathing while exercising. Most people start mouth breathing as soon as they step onto the treadmill, so this might feel a little strange at first. However, you will soon notice just how much activity you are capable of with nasal breathing alone, even if you've never tried it before.

The key is to exercise at a pace that is challenging enough that you need to flare your nostrils, but not so challenging that you are making snorting sounds or popping your ears. Consider the first week or two the ramping up process in reviving the power of your nose. You will be surprised at how quickly it will adapt. While there are other tips in this section, I cannot overemphasize the power of exercising for unlocking the potential of your sinuses. In time, you will be able to do high-intensity interval training, sprints, and many other high-intensity activities breathing 100 percent nasal. Remember, nasal breathing provides a superior gas exchange due to its facilitation of functional breathing and a boost in circulation due to the nitric oxide that you will be inhaling with every breath. In addition to getting the most out of every breath, you'll lose less hydration, which is a vital component to athletic performance.

When Speaking, Singing, and Dancing

We often revert to mouth breathing when doing activities that require a quick inhale. I was a university professor for over a decade, and I remember coming home each day exhausted. What I didn't realize is that while I lectured, I was mouth breathing. Then, when I met with students, I was mouth breathing. And when I spoke to my colleagues in meetings, I was mouth breathing. This mouth breathing caused me to chest-breathe most of the day, bringing me into a stressed state. I wouldn't notice until I began my drive home, and then it would hit me. I was exhausted! It wasn't until I started to consciously take a moment to inhale through my nose while speaking that I realized I had more energy at the end of the day. At first it was an awkwardly long pause, but in time, it became automatic. Before long, the pause wasn't even noticeable because my sinuses became less obstructed the more I used them. As you begin your nasal breathing lifestyle, don't forget to breathe through your nose, even in those times when mouth breathing seems automatic.

Slowing Down to Speed Up

Many people get into breathwork because they want to practice deep breathing exercises, which feel amazing. They often begin practicing using mouth breathing for one reason or another and find it difficult to breathe nasally as fully or with as much speed as with their mouth. If you can relate to this situation, the best thing you can do is accept that you will not be able to breathe as hard at first and simply slow down until your sinuses adapt. Eventually you will be able to breathe incredibly fast and fully through your nose, and you won't miss mouth breathing at all.

However, if you just can't seem to make yourself do this all at once, at least switch to breathing in through your nose and out through your mouth for a while. Then, as inhaling through your nose becomes more comfortable, begin adding nasal exhales. Perhaps you can add a nasal exhale to every other breath at first, and then eventually you can do five breaths 100 percent nasal. Be patient but diligent. The goal is 100 percent nasal.

Mouth Taping at Night

This is one of the recommendations I get the most pushback on from clients early on, but after they do it for a week, they always come back to thank me. Many people breathe through their noses all day, but when they fall asleep, their mouths fall open and they mouth-breathe all night. This causes irritation in the bronchi, bronchioles, and alveoli. It also reduces one's CO_2 tolerance, leading to faster and more erratic breathing patterns. While nasal breathing throughout the day helps somewhat to keep this in check, nighttime mouth breathing can keep a practitioner from realizing their nose's full potential. It can also induce stress sleeping, which is a very real problem. Perhaps you are familiar: people who stress sleep might get eight hours of sleep in a night, but when they wake up, they still feel unrested. If this sounds familiar, try taping your mouth shut before going to bed at night to ensure that you don't mouth-breathe. Just a little tape will do. You don't have to use duct tape.

Caring for Your Air

It might be that you are unable to breathe well through your nose because you are habitually breathing poor-quality air. Sinuses often become inflamed when bombarded by very dry or cold air (or both). I recommend keeping the humidity in your home between 30 and 50 percent. More than 50 percent humidity can lead to mold, which can invite a whole host of problems. Going lower than 30 percent can cause irritation and inflammation in the sinuses, which can make it difficult to breathe. It is especially important to ensure that the place where you sleep has quality air since you will be breathing there for a third of your day. Air filters are helpful as well during allergy season and if you live in a home with a lot of dust.

Paying It Forward

If you are a parent, one of the best things you can do for your child is to encourage them to breathe with their nose. While humans tend to accumulate dysfunctions due to sitting in chairs and hunching over smart phones, reminding children to breathe through their noses at least helps to keep them breathing functionally. This helps them to avoid overbreathing, which can heighten their levels of stress over the years. If only I could go back in time and tell myself that much of my stress was caused by all my mouth breathing! While I have had many parents ask me about what breathing techniques are best for children, my most common advice is to reinforce nasal breathing. This one habit can help keep their philias healthy and less stressed without needing to sit and focus on timed breathing techniques, which they will often not practice until they are older.

Language Lab 8

Unless nasal breathing causes you pain or severe discomfort, make the decision to breathe nasally all the time from this point on. It might also be time to see an ear, nose, and throat (ENT) doctor if you believe that you have a physical obstruction to nasal breathing.

When you exercise, make a conscious effort to breathe through your nose. If you don't currently exercise and you are able to, find a movement practice that's right for you. Exercise is another thing that your philia needs to be its healthiest. When you exercise, maintain nasal breathing as long as possible. If you need to breathe through the mouth, begin with only exhaling through the mouth while still inhaling through the nose. If, after doing this adjustment, you still cannot exercise, either reduce your intensity for a while to let your nose catch up to the rest of your philia, or go ahead and mouth-breathe. However, try to avoid mouth breathing at all costs unless you are in a competition, and then do so only at the very end of your sprint or match.

> Continue practicing the Awareness Exercise for ten minutes per day, longer if you have the time and desire.

> Continue to check in with your breath mechanics and posture throughout the day. Look up as often as you can, keep your shoulders back, and try to flex your glutes as often as you

can. Simply stretching commonly shortened muscle groups and flexing commonly relaxed muscle groups can do worlds of good for your posture and therefore for your breath mechanics.

> Keep practicing your favorite techniques, being mindful of the subtle nuances that you can add to each message with the manner of breathing that you use in conjunction with the technique. When we first learn a language, it takes a while to get the accents and inflections just right. The reply you receive from your unconscious-self will help you to determine how well you are progressing.

11

Team Building

"Let's take the test again," insisted Manuel, clearly unhappy with what he had just learned. He looked around at the others in the group, all of whom were equally surprised. I had just given a carbon dioxide (CO_2) tolerance test to a group of martial artists, and Manuel, like so many serious athletes who score low on this test, was unhappy with his results.

I often find myself speaking to groups of athletes looking to get an edge. Their competitive nature inspires them to do even the most difficult and unpleasant things if it will mean that they will be able to perform stronger longer. However, this competitive nature also sometimes makes it difficult for them to accept when they first discover their weaknesses, even though deep down, they know that discovering weaknesses is the key to becoming the best athletes they can be.

Manuel had moved to the United States with the singular goal of becoming the greatest Brazilian jiu-jitsu competitor in the world. He was well-known in Chicago, where I was presenting that day, and much to his surprise, he had scored very low on a test that we will get to later in this chapter.

An athlete's relationship to carbon dioxide will determine one of the most powerful limiters to performance: the feeling of breathlessness. However, this is not something that only athletes must deal with. Every one of us has a relationship with this molecule, and our relationship with it affects the relationship we have within our philia. After practicing the techniques in this chapter, Manuel was able to increase his CO_2 tolerance, and so can you. We just need to take our unconscious-self to the gym.

Understanding the Process of Cellular Respiration

To begin to understand why natural breathing quickens or slows under different circumstances, first we need to learn about the process of cellular respiration, the process by which our cells produce energy via the aerobic pathway.

A simple explanation of cellular respiration begins with the mitochondrion, sometimes referred to as the powerhouse of the cell. During the process of cellular respiration, mitochondria ingest oxygen (O_2) and glucose to produce adenosine triphosphate, more commonly known simply as ATP. This ATP provides energy for our cells, and without it we would die. One of the byproducts of this process is the molecule carbon dioxide (CO_2), which, you might remember, is the gas that is exchanged for oxygen in the lungs during respiration.

The process of respiration is a never-ending exchange of O_2 and CO_2, monitored by chemoreceptors located in the brain stem. What might surprise you, however, is that the urge to breathe is not triggered by a reduction in the amount of O_2 in the blood. Rather, when the chemoreceptors in the brain stem detect an increase in levels of CO_2 in the blood, you will feel the urge to breathe. If you hold your breath right now, eventually you will notice the subtle, and then not-so-subtle, voice of the unconscious-self letting you know that it is time to breathe. If you hold long enough, your unconscious-self will take control of your breathing and force you to breathe. While we do have conscious control over breathing, the unconscious-self eventually will take control.

When we are stressed and our sympathetic nervous system becomes activated, this process is sped up to increase our energy levels for fighting or running from a potential threat, creating more CO_2 and therefore a greater urge to breathe. When this happens, we tend to breathe faster than normal. For most of human history, this extra energy was used to help us take action to physically avoid a threat, to hunt, or to fight. When the threat was eliminated, the sympathetic side of our nervous system would become less activated and our CO_2 production would decrease, naturally slowing the urge to breathe. However, in the modern world, chronic unchecked stress can leave us in a chronic state of sympathetic nervous system activation, which keeps us breathing faster than we should.

Of course, this faster breathing can put us into an even higher state of autonomic arousal because, as we have learned, faster breathing sends a message of stress. If this cycle is left unchecked, it can lead us to a heightened state of anxiety and even into a panic attack. This is just one more reason why it is important to maintain awareness throughout the day to infer what our unconscious-self believes about the situation. Do we really need to energize? If not, we should begin to speak by using some comforting and calming techniques, being mindful of the tone and inflection of where we are placing each breath.

However, if we try to force a slower pace than what we can tolerate, we will suffer from the feeling of suffocation due to increased levels of CO_2. This feeling of suffocation can cause an overwhelming feeling of panic and fear[1] because our unconscious-self believes we are suffocating. Consequently, the natural response is to activate the sympathetic nervous system in a major way to ensure that you have the strength to escape whatever is preventing you from breathing. When this happens, we create even more CO_2 as we ramp up energy production, causing the situation to get even worse.

Therefore, when practicing the techniques we discussed in the previous chapter, especially when in moments of stress, it is important to slowly increase the lengths of breaths to avoid this suffocation response, only gently challenging the urge to breathe as we go.

Carbon Dioxide Is Not the Enemy

While carbon dioxide might be considered a byproduct of the process of cellular respiration, it is not something that we could live without. Simply put, when CO_2 is low in the bloodstream, our red blood cells cannot deliver oxygen to our tissues. This is due to a phenomenon known as the Bohr effect, first described in 1904 by the Danish physiologist Christian Bohr. However, if we can tolerate higher levels of CO_2, our ability to release O_2 into tissues is increased, meaning that it is to our advantage to be able to tolerate having high levels of CO_2.

CO_2 is a vasodilator, meaning that it opens our blood vessels, allowing for healthy blood flow. So, increasing our tolerance to CO_2 not only allows our red blood cells to disperse oxygen to the tissues, it also opens the blood vessels, allowing these cells to travel where they are needed. When we have low levels of CO_2 (hypocapnia), we experience vasoconstriction and a reduction in oxygenation of tissues, and we are usually breathing faster than needed, which sends a distress message to activate our sympathetic nervous system. Sadly, this is a condition more common than most of us realize.

Overbreathing—When the Philia Needs Couples Counseling

The Language of Breath Philosophy is all about bringing your philia together to work as a strong team, which is the healthiest version of you. However, many philias around the world suffer from a bad relationship because of something that has become all too common in the modern world: overbreathing.

Overbreathing is a common breathing dysfunction that causes us to exhale more CO_2 than is appropriate given the situation. As with many modern issues, we can point to causes that are only possible in the modern world. When it comes to overbreathing, most of us begin at a young age due to something we all know and love, carbohydrates.

Have you ever eaten way too much carbohydrate-filled food and later found yourself breathing heavily, even though exercise is the farthest thing from your mind? This is caused by respiratory acidosis from eating excessive amounts of carbohydrates,[2] a common occurrence in modern diets. When we eat high amounts of carbohydrates or sugars, the levels of CO_2 are increased in our blood. This is picked up by the chemoreceptors in our brain stem, which causes us to breathe faster and harder than normal. For many modern humans, this happens so often that we can just get used to breathing fast. Just as we can train ourselves to breathe functionally, we can also unwittingly train ourselves to breathe dysfunctionally. When overbreathing becomes habitual, we overbreathe even when we don't need to, lowering our normal levels of CO_2. Over time, our brain stem becomes used to lower levels of CO_2, making it more sensitive. This means that your urge to breathe comes faster than normal, making your normal rate of breathing faster.

Overbreathing can lead to more overbreathing. As our CO_2 sensitivity increases, we tend to breathe faster. As we have already learned, the faster we breathe, the more stress we speak to our unconscious-self. We activate our sympathetic nervous system, putting us into a stressed state. This heightened state of stress often makes us breathe even faster, as our unconscious-self is preparing for a potentially dangerous situation. This begins a feedback loop. Before long, we notice that we are breathing very heavily, which scares us, making us breathe even faster, which activates our sympathetic nervous system even more, leading us to breathe faster, which scares us even more, which activates our sympathetic nervous system even more. This can lead to a panic attack and even passing out because CO_2 levels have dropped so low that brain oxygenation is low enough to lose consciousness.

While most people who overbreathe do not have panic attacks, they certainly carry around a higher base level of stress than necessary. As we discussed earlier, chronic stress causes an elevation in cortisol levels that, in time, can lead to increased inflammation, a weak immune system, and high blood pressure. This is not helped by the fact that overbreathers cannot take advantage of CO_2's vasodilation capabilities because they are constantly keeping their levels low. Simply put, a low CO_2 tolerance is the end result of overbreathing, making over-breathing a cause of major disconnection within one's philia.

The reduction in CO_2 levels in the blood has been shown to constrict blood vessels in the brain and the heart; reduce blood flow to the brain as much as 50 percent, reducing oxygen and glucose to the brain; and make brain cells become more excitable. Low blood levels of CO_2 have also been shown to constrict smooth muscles around the bronchioles, making breathing more difficult and less efficient.[3]

The good news is that with practice, you can improve your tolerance to CO_2 using a variation on The Awareness Exercise you already know, which I *hope* you practice every day whether you are using this variation or not.

Gym Buddies—Increasing CO_2 Tolerance to Make the Philia Stronger

When I was thirty, I finally began taking my health seriously. Up until that time, I was a mess. However, when I went to the gym with my friends who were already in good shape, they would always push me so hard that I dreaded going back. It wasn't until I was able to work out on my own that I was able to slowly increase the intensity of my workouts, which led to better overall results because rather than trying to make a ton of progress all in one workout only to lapse in my training and make no progress at all, I kept coming back every day. Real results are achieved by being diligent over time, not all at once.

I'm making this point to you now because you are about to take your unconscious-self to the gym. In this case, you will consciously create an elevation in your CO_2 levels that will cause your unconscious-self to respond with feelings of discomfort. It is up to you to ensure that you don't make the experience so uncomfortable that you just never train again.

When it comes to your philia, actions are the words. Just as we must challenge our muscles to make them stronger, we must also challenge our CO_2 tolerance to increase it. Before we begin, let's make sure your philia is ready.

How to Measure Your CO_2 Tolerance

The simplest way to measure your CO_2 tolerance is to perform the CO_2 Exhale Test. This is a common test used among athletes and breath trainers because it is hard to mess up. I picked it up from elite fitness trainer Brian Mackenzie. It involves taking the biggest breath possible and timing how long you can make the exhale last. Before taking the test, breathe normally. While you read the following directions, don't mimic the test; just breathe naturally to avoid getting an inaccurate score. You will need a stopwatch.

Step 1: Take a deep breath through your nose and relax it out to neutral lungs.

Step 2: Wait until you feel the urge to breathe, then take another deep breath and relax it out to neutral lungs.

Step 3: Wait until you feel the urge to breathe; then take a deep and full breath through your nose.

Step 4: Begin the timer as you exhale through your nose for as long and as slow as you can.

Stop the stopwatch when one of the following things occur:

1. You completely run out of air.

2. You swallow.

3. There is ever an interruption in the airflow as you exhale.

Your time is your score.

SCORES AND THEIR MEANING

0 to 20: Very poor CO_2 tolerance. If this is your score, you might need to retest the following day to ensure that it is accurate. Many people score very low when they are under a great amount of stress or they are sick. If this is your score, before training to increase your CO_2 tolerance, you need to improve your score to at least 20. I would recommend using cardiovascular exercise to improve your CO_2 tolerance, which is one of the best ways to naturally improve this score. You may also greatly benefit from Box Breathing or Bottom Triangle. If you jump into CO_2 tolerance techniques before you score at least a 21, you risk adding to your stress rather than improving.

21 to 40: Average modern human. This score means that you can directly begin the CO_2 tolerance techniques later in this chapter. You have a lot of room for improvement, so get ready to train!

41 to 60: Advanced. This is a healthy range to be in. You can still train much higher, but at this level, you generally have a relaxed and smooth breathing pattern and can slow your breathing down somewhat easily after exertion.

61 to 80: Elite. This is a very good score, and most people need to train regularly to get here. At this point, your natural breathing pattern is slow and smooth, and you rarely breathe more than you need. At this range, you experience increased resilience against stressors.

80 and above: Master. At this stage, you have become very comfortable with CO_2, and you are very resilient against stress.

A WORD ON CO$_2$ TOLERANCE TESTING

It is generally best to test your CO$_2$ tolerance first thing in the morning. This helps you to avoid the rise in CO$_2$ production caused by eating, drinking coffee, or experiencing stress. If you do choose to test at a different time of day, just be sure to wait an hour after eating, and always retest at that same time of day to get an accurate reading of your changes over time. Your CO$_2$ production will change throughout the day due to many factors. This will change the scores. It is best to look at your score as a general indication of where you stand, expecting a little variation each time you test.

Now that you have an awareness of your CO$_2$ tolerance, let's make positive change by training to improve your CO$_2$ tolerance.

>>>>>THE CO$_2$-FOCUSED AWARENESS EXERCISE

Quick Note: It is best never to practice CO$_2$ tolerance training right after a meal. Wait at least an hour to allow your food to digest and your CO$_2$ production to reduce back to normal.

In the CO$_2$-Focused Awareness Exercise, we will practice the exercise as we normally would, but we will reduce the volume in our breathing to allow for a mild CO$_2$ buildup. This will cause you to feel an urge to take a fuller breath, but if you can calmly resist this urge, maintaining the higher levels of CO$_2$ for the duration of the exercise, you will challenge your unconscious-self to accept that CO$_2$ can be tolerated in higher amounts, raising your CO$_2$ tolerance. It is important to remember that, while you feel a mild sensation of suffocation, this is an illusion. You have plenty of O$_2$ in your bloodstream. You are simply allowing CO$_2$ levels to rise, which triggers the breathing urge. If you want to confirm this, you can purchase a pulse oximeter from any drugstore and test for yourself.

1. **Begin the Awareness Exercise as normal.** In the beginning it is especially important to practice this in a place without any distractions.

2. **Inhale, focusing on every part of the inhale.**

3. **Exhale, focusing on every part of the exhale.**

4. **Pause with a neutral-lungs apnea, focusing on internal awareness.** Allow yourself to practice the regular Awareness Exercise for a minute or two, becoming fully aware of your internal state, just as you would normally.

5. **Reduce the volume of each breath.** After a minute or two of normal practice, reduce the volume of each breath without changing the speed of your breathing, using the least amount of the breath wave as possible. Your goal is to breathe with as little of the breath wave and with as little volume as possible without feeling an air deficit. When you find this place, stay here about one minute. We are looking for the very edge of feeling an air deficit.

6. **Reduce the volume of your breath by just a little to create the feeling of an air deficit.** At first, this will be difficult to gauge, but with practice you will get it. The trick is to go very gradually into the air deficit rather than making a big change. It takes just a little while for the blood gases to resettle to the new level. Even if your air deficit is very mild in the beginning of this exercise, you will notice that after about a minute it becomes a little stronger. Stay calm and breathe as smoothly and gently as possible.

7. **Continue practicing the Awareness Exercise, reminding yourself that you are completely safe.** As you practice this variation of the technique, remember that you are coaching your unconscious-self to be comfortable with the sensation of breathlessness. This is best done gently. You don't want to push too hard. The goal is to create a regular routine that will progress with time.

If you accidentally come out of the air deficit, don't worry. Just gently drift back into it, remembering that this is a practice, not a performance. You will improve your skill, but you'll always be practicing. The power in the practice is diligence.

8. **Maintain the air hunger while practicing the Awareness Exercise for at least ten minutes.** While you can practice the CO_2-Focused Awareness Exercise for as long as you like, for marked improvements, a typical session should last approximately ten minutes. Does this mean a five-minute session is a waste of time? Of course not! However, challenge yourself to ten minutes as often as possible. To speed your progress, you can do multiple sessions throughout each day. **<<<<<**

Other Techniques for Improving CO_2 Tolerance

Ultimately, any technique that helps you stay calm while maintaining a mild urge to breathe will help your philia to become more CO_2 tolerant. The following techniques are favorites among most practitioners.

Edge Breathing

It usually takes around a minute for blood gases to find their new level, so what feels like a manageable urge to breathe at the beginning of a session might grow into an overwhelming urge to breathe if you start too ambitiously. Therefore, we always begin a CO_2 tolerance training session by "finding the edge." This simply means that we enter the session with a minute or two of practicing the technique at a pace and volume that is right at the edge of feeling a breathing deficit. We try to stay on that edge for about a minute before reducing the volume of breath. This helps to calibrate our training experience and leads to a more productive training session.

Edge Breathing is something you can practice throughout the day and when doing any of the ANS techniques you learned in the previous chapter. It is simply a way of breathing for your actual needs in the moment rather than overbreathing.

CO_2-Focused Balanced Breathing

Balanced Breathing is simple and easy to apply to CO_2 tolerance training. When we use a cadence of 5,0,5,0 we can combine CO_2 tolerance training with heart rate variability training. It is the easiest and most straightforward technique to apply to CO_2 tolerance training.

Instructions for CO_2-Focused Balanced Breathing

1. With a neutral spine, inhale through your nose for five seconds, using the least amount of the breath wave as is comfortable.

2. Exhale through the nose for five seconds, relaxing the breath.

3. When you have felt the edge of a breath deficit for a minute, decrease your breath volume slightly.

4. Maintain a mild breath deficit for ten minutes using this technique.

CO_2-Focused Balanced Breathing is a Language of Breath Philosophy staple because it makes finding the edge of a breath deficit easy for more practitioners.

CO_2-Focused Bottom Triangle Breathing

Bottom Triangle can be helpful for those who want to make sure that their breath speed is not changing. While the CO_2-Focused Awareness Exercise essentially involves all the same elements as Bottom Triangle (an inhale, an exhale, and a pause), it does not have to be done to a specific time, which can lead some practitioners to unwittingly adjust their breathing speed to accommodate for the lower breath volume, defeating the purpose of the exercise. Using a metronome and counting off your time is a safeguard against our tendency to compensate. The times should be 4,0,4,4 or longer, and your goal should be to begin the exercise using the lowest volume that you can without causing an air deficit.

Instructions for CO_2-Focused Bottom Triangle

1. Using a neutral spine and a minimal breath wave, inhale for four seconds.

2. Exhale for four seconds to neutral lungs.

3. Hold a neutral-lungs apnea for four seconds.

4. Repeat steps 1 through 3 for at least one minute.

5. When you have felt the edge of a breath deficit for a minute, decrease your breath volume slightly.

6. Maintain a mild breath deficit for ten minutes using this technique.

A WORD ON BOTTOM TRIANGLE FOR CO_2 TRAINING

The neutral-lungs apnea is an opportunity for CO_2 levels to rise, and without discipline this can get out of control. However, many practitioners find that the neutral-lungs apnea helps them relax in this exercise. This is a very important component of CO_2 tolerance training; use whatever helps you relax in the face of the stress of CO_2 buildup.

Big Bottom Triangle Breathing

Some practitioners practice a variation of Bottom Triangle known as Big Bottom Triangle, practiced using a cadence of 4,0,4,8 or greater. Using this technique, you can increase the intensity of the urge to breathe from mild to medium, increasing the challenge of the exercise. This will usually also increase the speed of progress, but remember that intensity should not come at the cost of consistency.

Instructions for Big Bottom Triangle Breathing

1. Using a neutral spine and a minimal breath wave, inhale for four seconds.

2. Exhale for four seconds to neutral lungs.

3. Hold a neutral-lungs apnea for eight seconds.

4. Repeat steps 1 through 3 for at least one minute.

5. When you have felt the edge of a breath deficit for a minute, decrease your breath volume slightly.

6. Maintain a mild breath deficit for ten minutes using this technique.

This variation of Bottom Triangle requires some skill and should only be practiced after one has practiced the CO_2-Focused Bottom Triangle technique. The extended neutral-lungs apnea can cause the feeling of breathlessness to increase to a more challenging level. This is fine if you can sustain it and remain calm.

CO_2-Focused Ratio Breathing

Because elevating levels of CO_2 stresses the unconscious-self, for many using a ratio cadence can be a helpful way to reassure your unconscious-self that things are okay. This can be done in the same way. The ideal cadence for most practitioners is 4,0,8,0, but this can be adjusted depending on your comfort level.

Instructions for CO_2-Focused Ratio Breathing

1. With a neutral spine and using the least amount of the breath wave as possible, inhale through your nose for a count of four.

2. Exhale slowly for a count of eight.

3. Repeat steps 1 and 2 for at least one minute.

4. When you have felt the edge of a breath deficit for a minute, decrease your breath volume slightly.

5. Maintain a mild breath deficit for ten minutes using this technique.

Many find that the difference between the inhale and exhale makes Ratio Breathing difficult to use for CO_2. However, it is worth trying, especially if you want to train CO_2 tolerance during times of heightened anxiety in your life.

Building Your CO_2 Tolerance Training Program

While there is no "perfect" CO_2 tolerance, higher is generally better. However, you only have so many hours in a day. Let the following program be a guide to get you started.

Upon rising:	Ten minutes of the CO_2-Focused Awareness Exercise
Mid-afternoon:	Ten minutes of any CO_2-focused technique you like
Before bed:	Ten minutes of the CO_2-Focused Awareness Exercise

To enhance this schedule, practice Edge Breathing when walking. You can also add extra sessions. While there is no limit to how much time you can dedicate to CO_2 tolerance training, my advice is to spend no more than a total of an hour each day focused on CO_2 tolerance exercises.

Athletic Training CO_2 Protocols

Everyone should desire to improve their CO_2 tolerance, but no group benefits more from this than athletes. People with high CO_2 tolerances are more resilient to stress, have better circulation, and have improved oxygen delivery to tissues, and this can translate into significant improvements in endurance and performance.

When athletes with high CO_2 tolerance step onto the field of play, their breathing is naturally slower because the CO_2 trigger to breathe is delayed. This creates a calm tone and presence within the philia, leading to a lesser degree of autonomic arousal. In everyday language, this means that while athletes with high CO_2 tolerance might have pregame jitters, their breathing patterns will be less likely to add to their stress, allowing the athlete to arrive to the competition calmer and more relaxed, avoiding the common pregame or early-game adrenaline dump that can lead to sluggish performance in the latter half. This calmness puts the athlete in a state where creative thinking is more accessible, leading to fewer errors.

CO_2 production increases during physical exercise. In a dead sprint, a philia with high CO_2 tolerance will be able to push stronger for longer before succumbing to being "out of breath," and the higher levels of CO_2 that this philia will be able to tolerate will provide for improved circulation and oxygen delivery to tissues.

When the sprint is done, athletes with high CO_2 tolerance will be able to "catch their breath" faster because their edge of breathlessness will have moved to accept a higher CO_2 level in the blood. This reduced recovery time places them in a better state for the next round. Athletes who compete in sports where there is heavy exertion separated by short breaks will enter the subsequent exertion more recovered than their competitors.

Post competition recovery begins faster for CO_2-trained individuals because breathing returns to normal faster and is more likely to be slow and relaxed during the day, leading to a natural state of recovery (parasympathetic).

How to Get the Athletic Benefits of CO_2 Tolerance Training

While the techniques described in the first part of this chapter will improve CO_2 tolerance, athletes will also need to train while moving to see the fullest benefits of CO_2 tolerance training. This can be done as simply as adding walking, running, or rowing to any of the exercises described in this chapter. Below are some examples of how one can apply techniques to physical training.

Instructions for CO_2-Focused Balanced Breathing While Walking

1. Begin walking at a pace of one step per second to help you keep time.

2. Inhale through your nose for five seconds or five steps, using the least amount of the breath wave as is comfortable.

3. Exhale through the nose for five seconds or five steps, relaxing the breath.

4. Reduce the volume of your breaths to find the edge of an air deficit.

5. When you have felt the edge of a breath deficit for a minute, decrease your breath volume slightly.

6. Maintain a mild breath deficit for ten minutes using this technique. After ten minutes, return to Edge Breathing without gasping or taking a big breath.

7. Try to breathe at the edge of a breath deficit until you are done with your walk or until you decide to do another ten minutes of CO_2-Focused Balanced Breathing during your walk.

The intensity of this exercise can be increased by walking faster. Remember that increasing your physical activity will increase your CO_2 production, which will increase the challenge of this exercise. Increasing the intensity of the urge to breathe can increase your results faster. Just be sure to keep your breathing cadence and volume unchanged, and don't forget that persistence is the most important factor.

Instructions for CO_2-Focused Top Triangle While Running

1. Begin running at a consistent pace, using your steps or an audio track to help you keep time. Try to maintain a consistent pace.

2. Inhale through your nose for four seconds, using the least amount of the breath wave as is comfortable. A full breath is completely fine.

3. Hold with your desired fullness for four seconds.

4. Exhale through the nose or mouth for four seconds, relaxing the breath.

5. Reduce the volume of your breaths to find the edge of an air deficit.

6. When you have felt the edge of a breath deficit for a minute, decrease your breath volume slightly.

7. Maintain a mild breath deficit for ten minutes using this technique. After ten minutes, switch to Edge Breathing (at a natural cadence, just monitoring your breath volume) without gasping or taking a big breath.

8. Try to breathe at the edge of a breath deficit until you are done with your run or until you decide to do another ten minutes of CO_2-Focused Top Triangle during your run.

Instructions for CO_2 Bottom Triangle While Rowing

1. Begin rowing at a consistent pace, using your pulls to help you keep time. The goal is to be consistent with your pace.

2. Inhale through your nose for four seconds, using the least amount of the breath wave as is comfortable. A full breath is completely fine.

3. Exhale through the nose or mouth for four seconds or four pulls, relaxing the breath.

4. Hold with neutral lungs for four seconds. Reduce the volume of your breaths to find the edge of an air deficit.

5. When you have felt the edge of a breath deficit for a minute, decrease your breath volume slightly.

6. Maintain a mild breath deficit for ten minutes using this technique. After ten minutes, return to Edge Breathing (at a natural cadence, just monitoring your breath volume) without gasping or taking a big breath.

7. Try to breathe at the edge of a breath deficit until you are done with your session or until you decide to do another ten minutes of CO_2-Focused Bottom Triangle during your rowing session.

The previous three CO_2-focused sessions are just examples of what can be done. Steady exercises such as walking, running, or rowing are ideal for CO_2 tolerance training because they can be done at a steady pace. When applying exercise to CO_2 training, ideally your breath volume will be the only variable that changes to create the CO_2 training stimulus associated with an increased urge to breathe. So, doing this kind of training while playing basketball or tennis is possible, but it is difficult to manage due to the changes in physical exertion that are associated with these activities. If you still want to try, I recommend practicing Edge Breathing for these activities, which will still engage your CO_2 tolerance in a challenging way.

Building Your Athletic CO_2 Tolerance Training Program

Again, you will need to experiment to determine what works best for your life and training goals, but the following is a sample daily schedule for those wanting to enhance athletic performance.

Upon rising:	Ten minutes of the CO_2-Focused Awareness Exercise
Main exercise session:	Three sets of ten minutes of any CO_2-focused technique you like while walking, running, or rowing, using two to five minutes of Edge Breathing between sets
Mid-afternoon:	Ten minutes of any CO_2-focused technique you like while walking
Before bed:	Ten minutes of the CO_2-Focused Awareness Exercise

To enhance this schedule, practice Edge Breathing when walking throughout the day. You can also add extra sessions as desired.

Testing and Retesting

Test your CO_2 tolerance as often as you like. At first, you will notice improvements in your CO_2 tolerance scores relatively quickly, so daily testing will be quite exciting. Eventually, you will begin to find your peak CO_2 tolerance. Yes, there will be a point where you cannot increase your CO_2 tolerance. This is part of being a human being. At that point, most practitioners check their CO_2 scores periodically. It's up to you, but don't obsess over numbers. Just stay true to your training.

CO_2 Tolerance and Taking Action

With an increased tolerance for CO_2, you are more resilient to stress. This means that you will be able to tolerate higher levels of stress before becoming overwhelmed. This is good for a lot of reasons, but chiefly among them is that the greater your resilience to stress, the greater your ability to think and make decisions under pressure. Life is going to throw situations at you where your ability to act appropriately under pressure will change the outcome, possibly with big consequences. Taking your unconscious-self to the CO_2 gym not only improves your ability to take physical action; it can also help you keep your calm.

Language Lab 9

As you build your inner relationship, consider dedicating time for CO_2 tolerance training. Using the information in this chapter, you can strengthen your philia, not only enhancing the effectiveness of the techniques that you choose to employ but every breath you take as well.

> Continue to use techniques as phrases, feeling free to create your own using what you learned in chapter 9. Experiment

with practicing techniques in a series to enhance your communication with your unconscious-self. Remember that how you breathe the techniques will play a great impact in how your messages are received. The technique is the phrase, and the way you breathe is the tone and presence. This can take a lifetime to master, so don't be frustrated if you progress slowly. However, don't waste time just going through the motions either.

> Continue to practice the Awareness Exercise for ten minutes or more per day. Feel free to add CO_2 tolerance training to this practice, but also reserve some time for the original practice and the Advanced Awareness Exercise. The CO_2 focus will make it difficult to observe yourself and how thoughts affect your philia. It's important to have some time just to continue to work on developing internal awareness.

> Continue using your nose all the time, checking in with your breath mechanics and posture often throughout the day as well.

12

Superventilation, Circular Breathing, Hypocapnia, and Bliss

Many people find breathwork by way of a technique that involves hyperventilating on purpose. This style of breathwork goes by many names. Some call it "voluntary hyperventilation." I prefer using the term "superventilation" for any instance where you are breathing faster than you need to on purpose. Regardless of what you call it, breathing fuller and faster than you normally would is another way to send messages to the unconscious-self.

In normal circumstances, breathing fuller or faster than your immediate needs demand is a bad idea. We just discussed the negative consequences of overbreathing regularly and how it can cause a cascade of adverse effects due to the effect of overbreathing on CO_2 tolerance. However, superventilation, when practiced responsibly and with respect to the effects on the philia, can be a beautiful addition to your practice and inner relationship.

Superventilation activates the sympathetic nervous system and reduces the amount of CO_2 in the blood. Sympathetic activation has been shown to activate the release of endogenous opioids, which can reduce pain and create a pleasant feeling; prolonged reduced levels of CO_2 (hypocapnia) have been shown to induce altered states of consciousness.[1] Superventilation techniques have also been linked to creating a state of "flow" or "being in the zone." This combination has made superventilation very popular—and unfortunately often overused, abused, and misused.

However, when used responsibly and appropriately, superventilation can be a wonderful way to break out of ruminations, improve overall health, and simply feel good. In this section, we will cover the ways that you can use superventilation to bring about bliss and a stronger philia while avoiding the pitfalls that are common in the world of breathwork. However, before continuing, please see the "Health Considerations" section at the end of the book. It covers health contraindications to ensure that you will be doing your philia a favor and not a disservice, especially if you suffer from cardiovascular-related illnesses.

Within the Language of Breath Philosophy, we practice superventilation for the following reasons:

1. For immediate relief in times of emotional and physical overwhelm.

2. To break out of rumination and overthinking to help us avoid being stuck in a fear-based state of inaction.

3. To provide an opportunity to strengthen our philia by way of hypoxic training.

4. To increase creativity.

5. To feel good.

In addition to these five goals, which are covered in this chapter, we will also use a kind of superventilation in the next chapter, where we focus on connecting to our unconscious-self on an emotional level, providing a way to make life choices more aligned with what we really want deep down.

Taking Smart Actions in Times of Overwhelm

We understand that our unconscious-self is always trying to help us survive and thrive, but this can bring with it a great feeling of overwhelm in many situations. It is often these times when we are called to make clear and concise decisions and act in ways that can have positive or negative repercussions depending on our ability to think logically and creatively. In these situations, we usually call on our ANS techniques to speak calm and balance into our philia.

However, if you have a moment to yourself in times of overwhelm, the following technique can alleviate some of the CO_2 build-up that can come with intense emotional and physical stress and it can provide a way to reset your outlook. I call these the times when we must be "the adult in the room." For instance, I always teach this in my first responders programs. We ask these individuals to oversee potentially traumatizing situations daily, and we still expect them to be able to operate professionally and with poise. While I instruct them to always use every breath to speak calm into their philias, I also teach them the following technique to use in the few moments when they are not directly engaged.

Practicing the Sniff Sniff Poo Technique

The Sniff Sniff Poo Technique is one of the only techniques that allows for the option of exhaling through your mouth. Sometimes, when emotionally overwhelmed, our noses get stuffy. While this technique is just as effective using 100 percent nasal breathing, when the goal is to speak peace into your philia during times of overwhelm, just do what is easiest for you.

The Sniff Sniff Poo Technique gets its name from the sounds that you will make when practicing it. Before you try this technique, use your sense of internal awareness to take account of how you feel. Apply the skills you have learned by practicing the Awareness Exercise to be fully aware as you practice the technique and after.

Instructions for Sniff Sniff Poo

1. In a seated position with a neutral spine, using the breath wave in the proper order, inhale to 70 percent full lungs through your nose.

2. After pausing for only a moment, fill the rest of your lungs by inhaling through the rest of the breath wave to the fullest lungs you can.

3. Exhale through your mouth making a "poo" sound with your lips.

This technique can be used just once, or it can be repeated as needed. Try it just once first, then assess how it makes you feel. When you have become aware of how one repetition feels, move to the next section.

A Sniff Sniff Poo Session

Remember to use your sense of awareness before, during, and after this session. We are looking for peace that we can take with us for the purpose of engaging the situation to make positive actions. We aren't trying to escape.

1. Come to a seated position with a neutral spine. Using the breath wave in the proper order, inhale to 70 percent full lungs through your nose.

2. After pausing for only a moment, fill the rest of your lungs by inhaling through the rest of the breath wave to the fullest lungs you can.

3. Exhale through your mouth making a "poo" sound with your lips.

4. Repeat ten to thirty times.

5. Return to normal breathing, but try to breathe as slowly as comfortable, allowing yourself to become aware of the peace that this moment can offer, despite whatever it is that you are going through.

You can repeat this protocol up to three times. Then go back to the situation with newfound peace to help you act with a positive outlook.

Using Sniff Sniff Poo after Physical Exertion

Sniff Sniff Poo is also very useful in times when you are experiencing CO_2 build-up due to physical exertion. Whether you are an athlete or on a weekend hike, this technique helps to open alveoli and clear out excess CO_2. While I would ultimately encourage you to try to tolerate the built-up CO_2 to help reinforce a high CO_2 tolerance, in extreme situations, CO_2 buildup can cause you to experience anxiety and reduce your ability to think clearly. In these instances of physical overwhelm, just as with emotional overwhelm, if you still need to keep your cool in order to make better decisions, go ahead and use Sniff Sniff Poo to bring yourself back into a state where you can think more clearly.

Interrupting Rumination

We know that messages are always being sent within our philia; however, it is common for humans to ruminate and overuse their conscious thinking. We often refer to this as being "too in our thoughts" or "stuck in our heads." Our unconscious-self, trying to help encourage us to consciously take action to solve the problem or eliminate the uncertainty around it, will continue to feed us dopamine. This can cause us to ruminate, to consciously think of more reasons to worry, which leads the unconscious-self to send even more dopamine and other stress hormones to help us to act or think critically to solve the problem. This can lead to a feedback loop that can make us so anxious that we lose our ability to think creatively and positively. Sometimes we need to interrupt our inner dialog to refocus and to take action in positive ways.

When we are lost in rumination and overthinking, we often fail to take actions that will improve our lives. Remember, as a human, your survival strategy is about taking action. While the world around us has changed, this foundational attribute of being a human has not. Whether you need to take actions to improve your health or your employment situation or whether you are having trouble getting up the nerve to talk to people to make friends, life is about taking action.

Still, sometimes we simply cannot act on the things that are causing us to ruminate. A common problem is that we become so engrossed in worries about which we cannot take action that we become paralyzed, letting other things slide. This creates a snowball effect. Before we know it, not only are we stressed about the thing that we can't change, but we also have created even more reasons to be stressed due our inaction.

In these times, a Sniff Sniff Poo session is a great choice. Another protocol that you can use is the Interruption Protocol. This protocol uses two speeds of circular breathing followed by three Peaceful Apneas.

For this protocol we will be using circular breathing, which is just another way of saying that there will not be any pause between inhales and exhales. We will breathe at a cadence of 4,0,4,0 at first, then move to 2,0,2,0 inhaling through the complete breath wave in the order of belly, ribs, chest on the inhale and relaxing the breath wave in the order of chest, ribs, belly on the exhale. While every inhale will be as full as possible, you do not need to forcefully exhale. Just relax the exhale and allow the natural recoil of the lungs and the relaxing of each muscle group to do the work. You will have neutral, not empty, lungs at the end of each breath.

All of this will be done with nasal inhales and nasal exhales. If you have not become able to do 2,0,2,0 using the nose only, remain breathing at 4,0,4,0 until you can go faster. In the worst-case scenario, if you cannot breathe nasally at a pace of 4,0,4,0, you may exhale through the mouth until you have developed yourself enough to be 100 percent nasal.

The Interruption Protocol

Following the circular breathing, this protocol calls for three Peaceful Apneas. See the instructions for how to do Peaceful Apneas at the end of chapter 9.

Now let's put it all together into a single breathing protocol.

Instructions for the Interruption Protocol

1. Lying down or in a seated position, begin breathing at a cadence of 4,0,4,0.

2. Stay at the 4,0,4,0 pace for one minute, focusing on using the breath wave to its fullest capacity.

3. After one minute at 4,0,4,0; speed up to 2,0,2,0.

4. Breathe at 2,0,2,0 for one minute.

5. After one minute of 2,0,2,0, perform three Peaceful Apneas, extending the exhale by humming or with a swishing sound.

6. Return to normal breathing and get started on doing an action that will improve your situation.

> **A WORD ON THE INTERRUPTION PROTOCOL**
>
> *The goal of this protocol is to put you into a better state. This protocol also feels really good. It is okay to do this protocol simply to feel good too. It doesn't just have to be in times of overwhelm. However, it is important to remember that excessive use of superventilation techniques can reduce your CO_2 tolerance.*

Hypoxic Training

When we overbreathe, we reduce the CO_2 in our blood. As we discussed in chapter 11, the urge to breathe is triggered by rising levels of CO_2 in the blood. One of the ways we can take full advantage of superventilation is to use this lowered level of CO_2 to allow for a longer apnea than we would normally be able to take. This is a way to induce intermittent hypoxia, which is a lowered level of oxygen in the blood.

Of course, low blood oxygen saturation (SpO_2) is typically a sign of underlying health concerns. This is why doctors will place your finger in a pulse oximeter when you visit their offices. On an ordinary day, blood oxygen saturation should fall somewhere between 95 and 100 percent. While this fluctuates during the day and can dip lower when doing intense exercise, this is the healthy range.

However, in healthy individuals, when practiced safely and deliberately, lowered levels of blood oxygen saturation have been shown to induce the production of the glycoprotein hormone, erythropoietin (EPO), which increases the oxygen-carrying capacity of the blood by increasing the number of red blood cells.[2] You might be familiar with the common practice of training at high elevations by elite athletes for the purpose of achieving this adaptation. The great news is that we can induce this process at sea level when we use superventilation to create a hypoxic state. However, there are more than just athletic benefits to the practice of hypoxic training. This is also an excellent opportunity to practice internal awareness.

Practicing Hypoxia-Focused Awareness

In the Hypoxia-Focused Awareness Exercise we cover momentarily, we will begin by practicing the Awareness Exercise as we normally would, bringing full awareness to our inhale, full awareness to our exhale, and using the pause between breaths to fully become aware of our philia from head to toe.

After two minutes of the standard Awareness Exercise, we will remove the pause between breaths, scanning the philia from the toes to the head in the inhale and from the head to the toes on the exhale.

Set your breaths to a cadence of 4,0,4,0 for one minute, then move to 2,0,2,0 for a second minute, inhaling through the complete breath wave in the order of belly, ribs, chest, and then relaxing the breath wave in order of chest, ribs, belly on the exhale. While every inhale will be as full as possible, you do not need to forcefully exhale. Just relax the exhale and allow the natural recoil of the lungs and the relaxing of each muscle group to do the work.

All inhales and exhales should be nasal. If you have not become able to do 2,0,2,0 using the nose only, remain breathing at 4,0,4,0 until you can go faster. In the worst-case scenario, if you cannot breathe nasally at a pace of 4,0,4,0, you may exhale through the mouth until you have developed yourself enough to be 100 percent nasal.

Neutral-Lungs Apnea and Breath Sips

After the two cadences of circular breathing are complete, you will take one last deep breath, allowing the exhale to fall out of your lungs to a relaxed neutral-lungs apnea. You will hold in this apnea for ninety seconds to three minutes. You will notice that you can hold this apnea for much longer than you could normally.

The goal of this apnea is to allow your mitochondria to use up the oxygen in your blood, reducing your blood oxygen saturation as significantly as possible. If you have a pulse oximeter, you can watch your SpO_2 drop below 95 percent, which signals the beginning of your hypoxic experience. With practice, you can reduce SpO_2 very low, often to levels as low as 40 percent. If it were any other time, this would be very dangerous, but doing it in a focused session such as this sends the message to the unconscious-self that you need to increase your red blood cell count to improve oxygen carrying capacity.

While the Hypoxia-Focused Awareness Exercise adds elements of time and the possibility of using a pulse oximeter to observe the drop in your blood oxygen levels, don't let these things get in the way of your internal awareness. If you have been practicing the Awareness Exercise, you should have developed your sense of internal awareness somewhat by now, so these added elements should not be a major distraction. However, if you find yourself watching the clock or the pulse oximeter more than observing your internal awareness, put them away. You can find a simple guided track to help keep you from focusing on the numbers too much at www.languageofbreathcollective.com /bookextras.

The goal is to hold for at least ninety seconds, which offers a significant amount of time for O_2 to be consumed by your mitochondria. This is an important time to use your sense of internal awareness. As your CO_2 levels return, you will slowly begin to feel the urge to take a breath. The more you can relax into this urge to breathe, the longer you will be able to hold, and the longer you hold, the stronger your hypoxic experience, which in turn strengthens your philia.

The key is to stay relaxed; don't struggle. If you find that you can no longer stay relaxed, you can take a quick and tiny sip of air with your nose to alleviate some of the built-up CO_2. After doing this, go back into the apnea for the duration of the ninety seconds. In time, you will be able to make it to ninety seconds easily. All of this is a time to use your sense of internal awareness, listening to your unconscious-self as your philia goes to the gym.

Following the extended neutral-lungs apnea, the protocol calls for three Peaceful Apneas. See the instructions for how to do Peaceful Apneas at the end of chapter 9. These help to keep your philia relaxed during this practice. As you perform these apneas, maintain full awareness and see if you can feel the rush of relaxation come over you.

Now let's put it all together.

NOTE *Be sure to practice the following exercise in a safe location where, if you lose consciousness, you will not hurt yourself. Sit or lie down on the floor for this session.*

Instructions for the Hypoxia-Focused Awareness Exercise

1. Begin the Awareness Exercise as normal, lying down or in a seated position. Inhale, focusing on every part of the inhale. Exhale, focusing on every part of the exhale. In the pause between breaths, focus on complete internal awareness.

2. After two minutes of the Awareness Exercise, begin breathing at a cadence of 4,0,4,0, scanning your philia from toes to head on every inhale, scanning from head to toes on every exhale.

3. Stay at the 4,0,4,0 cadence for one minute, focusing on using the breath wave to its fullest capacity.

4. After one minute at 4,0,4,0, speed up to 2,0,2,0.

5. Breathe at 2,0,2,0 for one minute.

6. After one minute of 2,0,2,0, take one last deep breath and exhale to a neutral-lungs apnea.

7. Remain in the neutral-lungs apnea for ninety seconds to three minutes, depending on your level of training. Use your internal awareness to observe your philia, and hold only as long as you can remain relaxed. If you have trouble making it to ninety seconds, take a tiny sip of air in through your nose and out through your nose and go back into the apnea until ninety seconds have passed.

8. After ninety seconds to three minutes, complete three Peaceful Apneas.

9. Repeat this protocol between three to five times, then go back into normal breathing.

A WORD ON THE HYPOXIA-FOCUSED AWARENESS EXERCISE

The most important part of this exercise, as with everything in the Language of Breath Philosophy, is awareness, the foundation of all positive change. There is a significant amount of bliss that can accompany superventilation, which is good. However, if you find that the feelings of bliss are preventing you from scanning your philia and feeling the physical sensations that accompany this exercise, you should either slow down your practice or shorten the time spent circular breathing by 50 percent or more. From this point, you can gradually increase speed or time of circular breathing, but only as long as you can maintain awareness.

While hypoxic training can improve athletic performance by increasing our oxygen-carrying capacity, it should always be paired with CO_2 tolerance training, which will ultimately garner the greatest benefits to athletic performance. Because this sequence is so pleasurable to perform, I often have no problem asking athletes to add it to their routines. However, without a high CO_2 tolerance, much of the benefit of high oxygen-carrying capacity is limited. Even if we have lots of O_2 in the blood, it does us little good if we are regularly overbreathing due to low CO_2 tolerance. A healthy CO_2 tolerance will ensure that the oxygen can be dispersed into the tissues when physically active.

> The higher your CO_2 tolerance, the longer you will be able to hold your neutral-lungs apneas, and this will result in a stronger hypoxic signal that will increase the effectiveness of the hypoxic training. While hypoxic training is a great way to strengthen your philia, CO_2 tolerance should take precedence over hypoxic training.

Exploring Creativity and Feeling Good

Practicing superventilation is a way of asking the unconscious-self to help your conscious-self to quiet down. It is theorized that superventilation can induce a state of mind known as transient hypofrontality.[3] This is sometimes called a state of "flow" or "being in the zone." It is characterized by unusually low activity in the prefrontal cortex of the brain and is often associated with deep states of meditation. When we engage in superventilation, we are essentially asking our unconscious-self to tell our conscious-self to hush just for a moment. This can allow us to get out of our own way and let the ideas and insights that the unconscious-self has to offer bubble up.

Much more research needs to be done on how superventilation enhances creative thinking. You can experiment on your own. In fact, in writing this book, I have taken many superventilation breaks. My favorite way to break up my workday is to do sessions of Sniff Sniff Poo. No matter what you do, if you want to allow yourself to come at a problem with a fresh point of view, give superventilation a try.

Superventilation for the sake of feeling good is also okay. Sometimes we just need a little dose of feeling good, simply for the sake of enjoyment. It is certainly better for you than drinking alcohol or doing drugs. Of course, as with all things that make us feel good, it is important to remember to be responsible. You are speaking to your unconscious-self with every breath, and superventilation, especially when done in excess, can invite a heightened state of autonomic arousal that can add stress to your day rather than release it. Anything can be abused. Remember that breathwork is language, not a cheap high.

Language Lab 10

At this point you have learned a lot. Practical application is going to depend on your daily schedule and what you would like to add into your philia. Remember that your team is your own. Use your sense of awareness to determine the direction that your team needs to go. What are things that you would like to do to improve your team, and how are you using every breath to maintain a presence that reflects the philia that you would like to have?

> Continue to practice the Awareness Exercise for ten minutes or more per day. This will always be part of your practice because you will always need to work on being aware of your internal state. Adding the CO_2 focus is an excellent way to challenge your philia to grow stronger, so I encourage you to add a CO_2-focused session into your day. However, always remember that the Awareness Exercise and the Advanced Awareness Exercise are essential.

> Vocabulary! Throughout your day, use the techniques we learned in chapter 9 to speak to your unconscious-self. Remember that the meaning of your message will be affected by how you breathe when performing the techniques. This means that, just like when you are learning any language, the more you practice, the more natural using your breath vocabulary will become.

> Tone and inflection! Remember that your tone and inflection will depend on how you breathe each breath, so refer back to chapter 7 if you need reminders on where to put your breaths and how functional breathing impacts the tone and inflection of what you say when you use a breathing technique from chapter 9. Use your nose all the time, checking in with your breath mechanics and posture often throughout the day as well.

> While it is optional, I recommend trying to add superventilation into your practice unless you have any of the contraindications. Experiment with practicing superventilation for each of the reasons stated in this chapter. Limit your superventilation practice to one quality session per day and no more for the first month of your practice.

> If you are working on improving your CO_2 tolerance, *always* practice CO_2 tolerance training before you practice superventilation or at a completely different time of day. Never practice superventilation before trying to improve CO_2 tolerance. It will weaken the CO_2 tolerance training.

13

Connecting to Emotions

It has been said that we ask for advice when we already know the answer in our hearts, but we are just too afraid to listen to ourselves. Who ever said it has to be this way? But the truth is that we are often faced with choices and situations in life where we have a hard time knowing what we really want. Still other times we aren't sure why we are not happy with what we know we should be very grateful for. No one said that being a human is easy, but later in this chapter, we will learn a very special technique unique to the Language of Breath Philosophy. It is a breathing technique known as the Listening Exercise, a powerful way of connecting with your unconscious-self.

The Biological Function of Emotions

To begin with, let's talk about emotions. Why do we have them? In the modern world, stuck in a mind-body paradigm, their purpose doesn't seem clear. If I am driving around this flesh robot, how does it benefit me to feel fear? Or shame? Or gratitude? Or pride? Science fiction movies often feature alien races who are devoid of emotions. Guided only with pure logic and reason, they seem to be free of many of the problems that we associate with the emotionality of humanity. But, of course, by the end of the story, we usually agree that while emotions are strange and obtrusive in many cases, our lives just wouldn't be the same without them, and we decide to take the good and even the bad ones.

However, emotions are more than just random add-ons to the human experiences; they are powerful messages from our unconscious-selves. By now, you know what your unconscious-self is most interested in; helping you to survive and thrive. And you might remember that our primary survival strategy as humans is to take action. Would you believe that emotions are complex and powerful ways that the unconscious-self speaks to us, guiding our actions and behaviors to survive and thrive within our environment and within our given culture?[1]

Emotions are powerful messages from our unconscious-selves that create changes in our physical expression in numerous ways by adjusting the cardiovascular, neuroendocrine, musculoskeletal, and autonomic nervous systems. When we experience these emotions on a conscious level, we call them "feelings," and while we experience emotional feelings, we also experience what we often call "gut feelings" or "feelings of the heart." These are all coming from a part of you that loves you and is always trying to help you survive and thrive: your unconscious-self.

In the case of gut feelings or feelings of the heart, we must remember that our unconscious-self is always learning, always finding patterns, even though we are not consciously aware. Sometimes we might have a gut feeling to pick one choice rather than another, despite having no idea why that choice seems better. This was demonstrated by Antione Bechara in a study conducted on participants who were asked to play a game of cards where they were given access to four decks: A, B, C, and D. Each participant's emotional state was monitored using skin conductance to determine emotional arousal. Participants in the study quickly developed gut reactions to avoid decks A and B to avoid losing money. As it turned out, these decks were stacked with losing cards before the game began, and without being able to explain why those decks were to be avoided, participants, guided by their emotions, quickly began to avoid them.[2]

One interesting case of the unconscious-self learning patterns and moving a person through emotional feelings was performed by the French physician Édouard Claparède on an amnesiac, someone who had no short-term memory. Every time he visited the woman, he would shake her hand and introduce himself, since she never had any memory of meeting him. One day, he pricked her hand with a needle when she reached out to shake. Of course, she recoiled in shock when this happened, but the next day, she had no memory of the event. However, the next day, when he reached out to shake her hand and introduce himself, she refused to shake his hand. She couldn't say why. She just felt a strong feeling to avoid his hand.[3] Even in the case of one suffering from amnesia, the unconscious-self learned and protected her via her feelings.

The unconscious-self speaks to us via emotions based on what it believes is best for us. This does not mean, however, that it is always right. While it is generally good to "listen to your heart," the unconscious-self only knows what it has learned. There are times when we are moved by our emotions to do things that are not good for us, and there are some emotional states that are not helpful, even though they are all coming from a part of us that is just trying to do its job, trying to help us survive and thrive. The same unconscious-self that sends you an emotional push to embrace someone who will be a good partner is the one that can send you an emotional push to punch someone in the face or cheat on your spouse. Your philia is a team, and this means that your conscious-self must pull its weight too. As with everything in the Language of Breath Philosophy, taking positive action in life depends on working with our unconscious side, and this always comes down to learning to listen.

In this book, we have learned that much of our suffering comes from a state of misunderstanding ourselves, thinking we are something that we aren't, and treating ourselves in a manner that reflects this misunderstanding. We also tend to do this with emotions. Since we don't always understand where they fit in our paradigm, we are often left wondering what to do with them. Some of us seem to be dominated by our emotions, unable or unwilling to let the conscious-self do its job of carefully examining whether or not our emotions and feelings are pushing us toward something that is right for us. Others, equally confused about our emotions, might try to completely disconnect from them, learning strategies to avoid feeling anything. Still others, still confused about what emotions are, might feel guilty for feeling a certain way, adding a whole new layer to our emotional confusion: feeling bad about feeling a way that we believe is a bad way to feel. All of this can cause us to try to avoid our emotions altogether.

Avoiding our emotions is neither beneficial to our philia or even possible. Deep down, they are still there, coloring our experiences and impacting our decisions. However, when we choose to realize that these emotions are coming from a place of love and self-preservation, influenced heavily by the patterns that our unconscious-self has picked up by our lived experiences, perhaps we can begin to see emotions more like what they really are. They are powerful messages from a part of us that loves us and is only doing its best to move us to actions that we believe are in our best interest. You don't have to be dominated by emotions, just like you don't have to avoid them. In fact, learning to engage with emotions can be the beginning of the healthiest and happiest years of your life.

Embodied Emotions

Where do we feel our emotions? In the old paradigm, we might wonder if emotions are in the mind or in the body. With our new view on what we are, a whole organism that is in a relationship with itself and the outside environment, we can answer the question this way: Emotions are felt physically when they are brought to conscious awareness.[4]

While this is backed with scientific evidence, we can experience this phenomenon now simply by replicating the study on our own. Follow the steps below to find out where you feel emotions when you bring them up consciously.

1. Begin with the Awareness Exercise. Take a few minutes to become completely aware of how you feel now, in this moment. Once you have a good grasp of the way you feel, you can contrast it against the way you feel when you bring other specific emotions to your conscious awareness.

2. After a few minutes of becoming aware of your current state, take about two minutes to bring up the following emotions. You can do this by thinking of things in life that cause you to feel these emotions.

Notice where you feel sensations within your philia. Maybe even point to these places as you focus on them.

- Jealousy
- Gratitude
- Anger
- Love

When you have completed this exercise, take a moment to ponder the possibility that the way you feel is not only affected by the emotions that you are consciously aware of but by those that you are not consciously aware of. For those of us who ignore or willfully disconnect from our feelings, this is a reality that we might think we are avoiding. However, even though you might not be consciously aware of your emotions, your unconscious-self is still sending them, trying to move your philia in the direction it believes is best. How many times have you looked back on your actions and felt like you had no idea why you did such a thing? Disconnection with your emotions doesn't make them go away; it simply handicaps your philia by creating a disconnected team.

Another thought to ponder is this: even though you thought of things to elicit specific emotions, it is likely that you felt more than one at once. You might have thought of something that you knew would make you angry, but at the same time it brought with it fear, self-doubt, and a whole host of other emotions that mixed to create the sensation that you felt physically in the moment. Perhaps other emotions were also present: perhaps you experienced signals about things that had something to do with other things that happened earlier in the day or that you are anticipating in the future. All of life is happening at once, and your conscious-self is only in charge of so much of what your philia thinks about. You could come back tomorrow and run the same experiment and find sensations in different places, even after thinking about the same things. This shows us two things: (1) emotions are subjective and (2) how we feel emotionally is an ever-changing blend of all the things our philia is concerned with at any given time.

While our conscious-self can scrutinize the messages of the unconscious-self, the unconscious-self has a very big say in what we think about and how we feel about it based on the world that we have been presented with throughout our life. This means that it is important to be mindful of the people, places, and things with which we surround ourselves. While we do not often realize it consciously, our unconscious-self is learning from the experiences we have in life, forming a model of what the world around us is like. If you are around people who lie a lot, it is likely that you will begin believing that people are generally liars and cannot be trusted. If you are normally around people who are generous, you will likely have a view of people that is more generous. It is not fully understood how far this goes, but it is likely that everything we expose ourselves to plays a role in forming our outlook in the world. And once we have this outlook, it is very difficult for us to see the world in any other way. This can create major impacts on our decisions based on the worldview that our unconscious-selves has created based on the inputs it has had.

I think we have all had the friend who is consistently unhappy with his life, no matter how well paid or appreciated he is at work or how loving his spouse or children are. We have also met the person who cannot seem to stay out of trouble, even though we know that deep down he is a moral person. Or perhaps we have the cousin who keeps going from one abusive relationship to the next as if she is seeking them out. Then, of course, there is the person who always seems to make the right decision, who is generally happy with his lot in life, and who seems to see the world as his oyster. Objectively, they are all living in the same world. However, their subjective experiences of this world are completely different. Their pattern-detecting unconscious sides began learning patterns about this world from the day of their births, and from that point on, built a model of the way the world works, and how to survive within it, on what they had learned. In the beginning of this book, we discussed that we often build our conceptions based on misconceptions. Misconceptions, even those that are fatally flawed, often remain in use because we cannot see the world in any other way.

Fortunately for you, you are not just a mind driving around a body. There is a team within you: a relationship; a philia. While we might unconsciously have useless, limiting, or even downright unhealthy beliefs about ourselves or the world around us that might be getting in the way of us living our best lives or taking positive actions, we can apply the Language of Breath Philosophy to build a better awareness of these emotions and how they manifest so that we can take conscious actions to reeducate our unconscious-selves. While it might be hard to understand how our unconscious-selves can send such uncomfortable or unpleasant emotions in the effort to keep us safe, knowing that they are coming from a place of love can give us comfort, and knowing that we can take actions to become more in touch with our emotions and therefore our unconscious-selves provides us with the foundation for making positive changes within our philia, which will translate into a healthier outlook on the outside world.

But first, we must learn to sit with these emotions. This can be very challenging because emotions are very powerful and can be unpleasant. We often avoid our emotions, even without meaning to. We are about to learn a powerful protocol to help us reconnect with ourselves. It provides a safe and effective way to listen to what the unconscious-self has to say without having to relive traumatic experiences or retraumatize the practitioner, which is common in many other forms of breathwork.

Awareness, the Foundation of All Positive Change

At this point, I hope you have been practicing the Awareness Exercise. This is a foundational exercise for the Language of Breath Philosophy because it provides a framework for developing interoception, the sense of internal awareness. Sustained mindful interoceptive attention has been shown to improve emotional awareness and aid in emotional processing in profound ways, leading to the processing of things we have held onto unconsciously but that still color every experience we have.[5] We are often unable to process emotions when they happen, and these unprocessed emotions can color experiences completely unrelated to the thing that caused the emotion.[6]

Emotional awareness allows us to be aware of what our unconscious-self thinks and believes about a given situation. However, it is often difficult to develop a high level of sustained awareness for long enough to really hear what the unconscious-self has to say. This is the purpose of the Listening Exercise.

The Listening Exercise offers you a safe and effective way to tune in and listen to what the unconscious-you has to say about any given topic, allowing you an opportunity to process these emotions and gain insight on how you feel unconsciously on the topic. This can be about anything: a traumatic memory, why you can't seem to be happy with a given situation, or which choice to make at a given juncture. They say we often ask for others' advice when deep down we know what we want; we're just too afraid to listen to ourselves. This ends today. Today we will listen.

>>>>>THE LISTENING EXERCISE

Note: For a more detailed theoretical framework of why this exercise works to facilitate safe and effective emotional processing, visit www .languageofbreathcollective.com/bookextras.

Please observe the health contraindications for this protocol under "Health Considerations" at the end of this book.

The Listening Exercise should only be done when you can dedicate time to it, and you should only practice this exercise in a safe, quiet place. Because this exercise can lead to profound insights and emotional release, be sure never to practice it when you are rushed or when you cannot dedicate your full awareness to the practice.

The Listening Exercise follows a carefully curated sequence of breathing and focus. Before we cover this sequence, let's discuss each component of this exercise.

Time of Practice

Limit yourself to fifteen minutes or fewer to get an idea of how this technique works and how it makes you feel. These sessions can bring up powerful emotions that can be jarring for some people, so reach out to a certified Language of Breath Breathworker to guide you through a longer session if you wish to go longer and deeper. Wait until you are accustomed to the Listening Exercise before doing longer sessions on your own.

Begin with the Awareness Exercise

Begin with the Awareness Exercise for between two and ten minutes. Become completely aware of your philia, paying special attention to keeping your focus on your internal state of awareness only. Do not skip this step. It lays the foundation for the Listening Exercise.

Focus on Two Things

Before the circular breathing begins, you will bring to your conscious awareness a specific thing that you would like to explore with your unconscious-self. This can be anything from a decision you need to make, a memory that you can't seem to get over, a fear that you have, the person you would like to be, and so on. Anything you want to check in on with your unconscious-self is fine as long as you can focus on it clearly. You should dedicate the entire session to this one thing.

Before the circular breathing begins, you will bring your conscious focus to that thing, and then you will observe how focusing on it elicits physical sensations within your philia. The more often you have practiced the Awareness Exercise, the easier it will be to detect and focus on these sensations. Remember that this is a practice, not a performance. Throughout this exercise, do the best you can to focus on your chosen topic and the physical sensations that accompany it. We will sustain this focus throughout the entire exercise. Your conscious focus on the topic you have chosen might drift, and these sensations might change throughout the session. This is normal, but try not to let your thoughts wander to unrelated topics. We will discuss this in more detail later in this exercise.

Balanced Circular Breathing

Only after setting your focus on your chosen topic, and the physical sensations that accompany it, will you begin the circular breathing portion of this exercise. Remember to keep your focus on your chosen topic and the physical sensations that accompany it. This might require even more effort to do at first. This is all part of the process.

The Listening Exercise uses circular breathing to the cadence of 3,0,3,0. For some people this feels fast, and for others it will seem slow. Use a click track or a metronome to help you keep time. Music is fine for keeping time, but try to avoid music that has lyrics or using multiple songs in a playlist. (For a free guided audio track of this session, go to www.languageofbreathcollective.com/bookextras.) While you will need to be mindful to keep this time in the beginning, eventually it will become a natural rhythm that you will do automatically as you focus on listening to your unconscious-self.

Listening, Observing, Receiving

Once the circular breathing begins, your goal is to maintain your two areas of focus (your topic and the physical sensations that arise) and to simply be receptive to whatever bubbles up to your conscious awareness. This can be in the form of sensations or feelings at first; however, after around eight minutes, unique insights tend to bubble up to conscious awareness. Sometimes there is a distinct feeling of knowing something that you always knew but, for some reason, you didn't realize that you knew it. Depending on the topic you chose to focus on, you might develop an understanding of where your feelings for this topic have come from. In other cases, the answer to the problem will suddenly appear in your conscious awareness.

After around fifteen minutes, it is not uncommon to have dreamlike visions. Often these visions tell a story or show a narrative. On other occasions, these visions might remind you of a memory that you have forgotten or one that you didn't realize you had connected with the topic you chose to focus on in the session.

In some cases, your session might bring up uncomfortable sensations or thoughts. In these cases, it is important to continue your session, maintaining your focus on these things, knowing that, as difficult as it might seem in the moment, these sensations are coming from a place of love, from a part of you that is always trying to help you survive and thrive. Approach these sensations with openness and curiosity, without judgment. Simply be open to whatever your unconscious-self is saying. By sustaining your interoceptive focus, you are allowing this emotion to become a part of your conscious awareness, no longer buried or coloring your outlook without your awareness.

If you are practicing alone, or if you are new to integrative breathwork, only go for a maximum of fifteen minutes. This technique is quite powerful, so if you choose to practice it for longer than fifteen minutes, have a certified Language of Breath Breathworker present to guide you. You can find a list of trained Language of Breath Breathworkers at www.languageofbreathcollective.com. Only go as long as you are able to maintain focus, and do not let this exercise become more about the pleasure it will bring than about listening to your unconscious-self.

The God Breathing Technique

God Breathing is how we will end the session. This is a breathing technique that calls for the longest, slowest, fullest inhale you can take until your lungs are as full as they can be, and then the longest, slowest exhalation all the way to empty lungs. Then you repeat this for two minutes.

Basically, you are going from absolutely full to absolutely empty lungs as slowly as you possibly can comfortably for two minutes. This is how we signal that we are closing the session. During this time, just be open to whatever comes to mind, allowing yourself to process the experience.

Another time when you can use God Breathing is if, during your session, you feel overwhelmed by the bliss or the intensity of your experience, or if you simply feel too tired to go on. You can fall into God Breathing for a little while to take a break. This should only be done if you feel the need. Otherwise stay with the breath cadence and keep your focus on your chosen topic and the physical sensations that accompany it.

Post-Session Processing

After two minutes of God Breathing, just go back into normal breathing, but spend as long as you need to allow yourself to process. During this time, many practitioners report having moments of clarity, creative insights, and inspiration. Allow yourself at least five to ten minutes for this processing, but take longer if you would like. Now that we have gone over all the parts of the Listening Exercise, let's cover the basic steps so you can have your first experience.

INSTRUCTIONS FOR THE LISTENING EXERCISE

1. In a seated or lying-down position, begin with the Awareness Exercise for between two and ten minutes. Become completely

aware of your philia, paying special attention to keeping your focus on your internal state of awareness only. Do not skip this step.

2. Begin thinking about your chosen topic.

3. Observe the physical sensations that come from thinking about your chosen topic.

4. Keep your focus on these two things for a few moments.

5. Begin circular breathing at a cadence of 3,0,3,0.

6. Maintain focus on your chosen topic and the physical sensations that accompany it while sticking to the 3,0,3,0 breathing cadence for up to fifteen minutes. After you become experienced, or if you are guided by a Certified Language of Breath Breathworker, go as long as you feel you need.

7. Close the session with God Breathing for two minutes, being open and receptive to anything that comes up.

8. Go back into normal breathing, allowing for plenty of time to process your thoughts and feelings.   <<<<<

Processing Your Experience

The Listening Exercise can be an incredibly profound experience, leading to new insights and connections that have been outside of your conscious awareness for some time. In most cases, processing is easy, and interpretation is obvious.

However, it is important to remember that no matter what comes up, it is coming from a place of love, and it is coming from you. It isn't an outside crazy boogeyman. When we practice the Listening Exercise, we allow ourselves to connect more fully to our unconscious-self, and occasionally this can create confusion or even bring up desires that we consciously know are either wrong or immoral. If this happens to you, remember that you are only listening to a part of yourself who is always trying to help you survive or thrive. It puts together a semblance of the world based on your lived experiences and the culture that you live in. And sometimes, your unconscious-self is flat-out wrong. If this happens, take comfort in knowing that you have learned something about yourself, and now that you have conscious awareness of this, you can take it into consideration when you take actions.

In the last chapter, we will also discuss some ways to use what we have learned in this book to help reeducate our unconscious-selves, although some unconscious beliefs and attitudes may be harder to change than others. Awareness is the foundation of all positive change. If you become aware of an unconscious belief or worldview that you do not consciously believe serves you, the simple act of becoming consciously aware of it is a huge step in improving the actions you take from this time forward.

Listening to Uncover Unconscious Beliefs

One way to discover how you really feel about something is to choose it as your chosen topic and practice the Listening Exercise. For instance, you might begin a session choosing the topic: the person you aspire to be. When you bring this to mind, try to visualize this future self. Try to be as specific as possible about what you would like to become. How do you talk? How do you interact with the world? What do you want to become? When you do this, you will also unconsciously have thoughts about this future self. Your unconscious-self might feel that this is unrealistic. Perhaps you unconsciously don't feel like you deserve to have such a life for some reason. Maybe unconsciously you are afraid to make the changes in your life that you know you need to make to achieve your goal. There might be a complex mixture of emotions that comes up.

This is good, even though it might be difficult to decipher. Why? Those beliefs were there anyway. At least now you are taking actions to bring them more to your conscious awareness. When we become conscious of our limiting beliefs—or our beliefs of confidence and desire—no matter what we unconsciously believe, we can begin to understand a little more about why we might act and feel the way we do when, in life, we might feel moved to act or behave a certain way. Awareness is the foundation of all positive change. When you become aware, you can begin to anticipate and appreciate the emotions that you feel in your life.

Remember, it is the job of your unconscious-self to process enormous amounts of information quickly to try to keep you away from disaster, but it is not always concerned with being 100 percent accurate. This is your job, conscious-you. When you become more aware of your unconscious beliefs about something, you can use your conscious thinking to think about it critically. Maybe unconsciously you feel that you could never start your own business or ask out so-and-so on a date. Take the time to listen to what your unconscious-self has to say, respecting the fact that it might be right, and that it is certainly trying to help you survive and thrive. But then add your conscious thinking to it too.

Maybe now is the wrong time to start a business. Or maybe it is the right time, but you acknowledge that your unconscious-self is just concerned about what will happen if your business fails. As with any relationship, compromise is generally the best strategy. Perhaps you could make a three-year plan to start your business, saving up money to satisfy your unconscious fears about putting your family out on the streets while working diligently toward building the business in your spare time. Yes, the internet gurus might scream at you, saying, just take the big jump! That might be the best move for them, and it might be the best move for you. However, in most cases, working in direct opposition to your partner (in this case your unconscious-self) is a recipe for disaster.

Maybe now is the time to ask so-and-so on a date. Or maybe now is the time to break up with your partner. Our unconscious beliefs about our interpersonal relationships often conflict with our conscious actions. Many people stay in relationships when unconsciously they know they shouldn't. On the other hand, many people might be experiencing feelings that have nothing to do with their mate while consciously believing their feelings are about their mate. It would be nice if the Listening Exercise provided a verifiable graph of all your feelings and emotions. I'm sorry. It doesn't. There is still some deciphering you will need to do. However, in my practice, many of my clients who had been struggling with relationship issues have found the Listening Exercise to be very helpful in creating clarity around how they actually feel, which has led to some people breaking up and others sticking together. In each case, while an emotional toll is to be expected in any breakup, clients report that they are convinced that they are doing what they really wanted to do.

You can use the Listening Exercise to help you gain clarity about how you feel about anything. Again, you won't get a neatly printed chart with numbers and words. But try this exercise and see for yourself. Every time you practice it, you've taken an action to connect with yourself in a very real way.

Listening to Make a Decision

Overthinking and rumination are common when a decision needs to be made. Your conscious-self can plan ahead and run simulations of what might happen if you take option A or B. Sometimes we get so overwhelmed that deciding is a dreadful thing. In times like these, we often simply don't know what we want to do. But our unconscious-self probably has an opinion on the topic that has been glazed over due to our excessive focus on conscious thinking. The Listening Exercise can be a big help in determining what you want to do. This is not to say that you should not consciously appraise the situation or think critically after you've done the Listening Exercise to get your unconscious opinion on the matter, however. The healthiest you is a team. In the case of decisions, we often ignore what our unconscious-self says. Take the time to listen.

Listening to Let Go

In many cases, we hang on to emotions when we do not have the time or capability to process them. In cases like these, sustained interoception (internal awareness) has been shown to be an effective way to process emotions.[7] However, this can be unpleasant and difficult to do for long periods of time. The Listening Exercise provides a pleasant way to do just that. By focusing on what you need to let go of, and the physical sensations that arise when this comes to mind, you allow yourself to sit with it in a new way, allowing yourself to process the emotions that come with it. We can't unwrite the past or change the way things are, but we can begin to let go of the suffering that we tend to carry around with us needlessly when we make the conscious choice to listen to what our unconscious-self has to say about it.

Overall, remember that while this exercise can be intense and profound, it is not magic. You are simply reconnecting on a deeper level with a part of yourself that you often either avoid or simply ignore.

Listening to Take Positive Actions

The healthiest you is a team. The more in touch you are with your emotions, the more in touch you are with your deepest beliefs, values, and desires. Sometimes these will point you in the right direction. Sometimes they are things you need to be aware of to try to help yourself avoid making poor decisions based on unhealthy unconscious beliefs.

Ultimately, the Listening Exercise is a way to reconnect and check in on a deeper level than we usually do in normal life. When you are connected to your unconscious-self, you can work better as the team you were born to be, more confident in your actions because you have allowed yourself to listen to yourself. For many of us, this might be the first time.

A WORD ON FREQUENCY AND INTENSITY

The Listening Exercise should be practiced no more than one time per day, and it should never be practiced with any more intensity than what is described here. The goal is to process emotions and possible trauma without inducing further emotional distress or trauma. Ideally, this is a session that you would be led through by a Certified Language of Breath Breathworker before doing sessions longer than fifteen minutes. Visit www.languageofbreathcollective. com for more information on finding a Certified Language of Breath Breathworker to work with you.

Language Lab 11

To get the fullest effect of the Language of Breath Philosophy in your life, unless you have one of the contraindications, begin practicing the Listening Exercise as described in this chapter at least once per week. You can practice it once per day, but no more than one time per day to ensure that you are not overloading your system.

Practicing the Awareness Exercise is essential to get the most out of your Listening Exercise experiences, so if you have been slipping on the Awareness Exercise, get back into it. If you've not been slipping, don't slip! You're doing great. Continue to practice the Awareness Exercise at least ten minutes per day.

You can practice a separate superventilation session on the same day as the Listening Exercise, but they should be in different sessions, hours apart.

If CO_2 tolerance training is something that you are interested in doing, keep it up! Just ten minutes per day can move the needle and make your philia stronger and more relaxed. Avoid practicing CO_2 tolerance training after superventilation or the Listening Exercise. It is best to train CO_2 before superventilation or at a separate time of day. Many people find bedtime to be a good time since the slow breathing can also be a message that the unconscious-self interprets as a call to relax.

Never stop breathing through your nose. Continue to check in with your breath wave periodically throughout the day and be mindful of your posture. Take corrective measures if needed.

As always, stay in the practice of being actively involved with your unconscious-self. Remember that it is important to set a positive presence with your breathing. Use your awareness to infer how your unconscious-self is feeling about your situation, while being consciously aware of the actions that you need to take, use techniques to communicate with your unconscious-self to keep the team in the best state for action.

14

Use the Language of Breath to Take Positive Actions

We have come a long way. We now have a better understanding of what we are. Rather than seeing ourselves as machine operators, we see ourselves more holistically as a relationship within ourselves and in relationship with the environment around us.

Humans have a survival plan based on taking action. That is what the unconscious-self is trying to help us do. However, sometimes we can't take action. In these times we need to be able to interrupt our unconscious-selves' persistent nudging so we can get some rest. In other times, we can move toward positive action, but we need to communicate some calm to our unconscious-self to ensure that the philia can perform at its best. This chapter will cover some suggestions on how to use the language of breath to communicate effectively with our unconscious-selves to ensure that our team operates at its best.

Remember, You Are a Relationship, Not a Machine

One thing that is constant in life is change. In the world of breathwork, there is often a focus on developing "the perfect daily routine." The intention is good, but it unwittingly relegates certain times of the day as times when you practice breathwork and then implicitly designates the rest of the day as times when you don't. It would make perfect sense if you thought of breathwork as inputting a code into your machine so you could set the dials and knobs to "have a good day" and just repeat that daily. But we know better.

Hopefully, after reading this far into this book, you have realized that there is never a time when you are not interacting with the world, which means that there is never a time when your philia is not working together to interact with your environment. Think of breathing as the way that you consciously interact with your unconscious-self as an active member of your team. It isn't about control. It's about working with yourself rather than against yourself, knowing that you are a species built for action. How is your philia set to take the most positive actions right now?

When you look at your day, look at all of it as time when you are working as a team with your unconscious-self. Every moment of every day, there are messages being sent within you; there is never a bad time to speak back to help the unconscious-you work to put you in the best possible state for positive action. Every breath matters. Which breath matters the most? The one you are taking right now. Then this breath. Then the next breath, and so on.

The most important thing you can do to create a healthy philia is to use your sense of internal awareness as often as you can. Check in with your unconscious-self. If you need to use your heart rate to gauge your autonomic nervous system activation, do it! But always remember to practice conscious awareness alongside this objective measuring device. Awareness is the foundation of all positive change. When you sense that you are too activated or not energetic enough for the actions you need to take in life, let your unconscious-self know.

This means that you might simply breathe with mindfulness of your presence and tone (breath mechanics), or it might mean that you need to take a ten-minute break to take a seat and do some Sniff Sniff Poo. Of course, maybe you are in a meeting with other people and your unconscious-self is uneasy about the possibility that you will mess something up and lose social status (which might get in the way of thriving or surviving); you can always do some Cadence of Bliss (4,7,8,0) quietly for a few repetitions while switching back to Box Breathing or Ratio Breathing to keep your calm. Your unconscious-self is always trying to help you, but you must be an active member of the team and let it know when it is creating too much activation or not enough.

Establishing Anchor Points

The better you get to know yourself, especially by practicing the Advanced Awareness Exercise (but also simply by regularly using your sense of interoception or internal awareness), you will begin to notice patterns emerge in your days. This is normally when people create routines around specific times of the day that are generally problem times or opportunity times to work on strengthening the philia. I prefer calling these "anchor points" rather than routines. An anchor is a temporary stationary device that can be moved when needed, and this is how to think about your daily anchor points. Let your life be what guides your practice, not a set routine.

You might choose to begin each day with some time that you dedicate to breathwork. However, always begin these sessions with the Awareness Exercise or at least with a few moments of dedicated internal awareness before going into a specific technique or sequence. While you might think that every morning is the same, the reality is that we are not machines (Yes, I'm going to repeat this all the way through the book to make it crystal clear!). Give yourself the freedom to use your morning session to speak to your unconscious-self. What does it need to hear today? You can use your awareness to determine how well you slept last night and think about the things that the philia needs to do in the day. Perhaps you have been holding a low level of anxiety about something; allow your awareness of it to determine your breathwork session. Don't just do the same thing every day—like a machine. There is no one technique that is perfect in every circumstance, just like there is no one phrase or sentence that can be said in every circumstance. What will you speak into your philia this morning? Make every session meaningful and be willing switch things up if your philia would benefit from something different each day. Let your awareness guide your session, not a preference for a technique.

Many people will add an anchor point to waking, before meals, pre- and post-exercise, and before going to sleep. In fact, research shows that just fifteen minutes of slow breathing before bed increases sleep quality and improves the overall restorative process.[1] However, in addition to simply using slow breathing, you now know multiple ways to speak calm and relaxation into your philia. Think about how those last minutes of each day might be used to speak calm and rest into your philia rather than checking your phone aimlessly for that same amount of time.

Overall, remember that the state of your philia is always in relationship to your environment, whether real or perceived. Your unconscious-self will always try to put the team in the best possible state to take action. It is up to you as the conscious-self to critically think about your situation and communicate with your unconscious-self to adjust if needed. This never ends, so as often as you can, become aware of your state and breathe in a way that helps the team take appropriate actions.

Making Better Choices and Taking Positive Actions

It is well documented that chronic stress can lead to a reduction in executive function, reducing self-control and leading to impulsive behaviors and life choices that we later regret.[2] Sadly, unless we take active measures to improve our relationship with outside stressors, we can find ourselves repeating destructive patterns that we would be much happier if we could leave behind.

One of the most common mistakes is to choose inaction over action. Yes, you want to avoid destructive and harmful actions, but as a human, your survival plan cannot be changed. You are a creature of action. The goal is to take positive actions rather than destructive actions.

Chronic unchecked stress often leads us to make poor choices. Sadly, this can become habitual behavior if you don't learn to speak peace into your philia. Eventually this habitual behavior might be such a part of your life that you don't realize that it is not just a poor way to deal with stress, it is causing more stress. Before you know it, this lack of good judgment that was caused by unchecked stress might have caused you to make negative habits in every corner of your life. If this is the case, the good news is that you are not stuck.

STEP 1. BE AWARE   Hopefully, you have been following along with all the Language Labs in this book. Your first goal is to become aware of your internal state. You should be practicing the Awareness Exercise every morning and checking in with your state regularly throughout your day.

STEP 2. COMMUNICATE REGULARLY When you are under stress, chronically or in specific moments, it is essential to use your sense of internal awareness to listen to your unconscious-self while simultaneously using every breath to reassure, calm, and relax your philia to the appropriate level of activation. We tend to make the worst choices when we are hyperaroused or when we let stress build up. When you leave stress unchecked, your unconscious-self will likely continue to ramp up your autonomic nervous system. The more sympathetic dominant you become, the harder it will be to think critically, creatively, or with kindness. Being aware of your state and communicating calm with every breath or with specific breathing techniques will help to keep you in a state where you can see more options available to you so you can take the actions that are the most beneficial rather than acting on impulse and out of desperation.

STEP 3. TAKE THE MOST POSITIVE ACTION POSSIBLE One of the most common problems we face when trying to take positive actions in our lives is dealing with the stress of taking that action, the fear of failure, and the overthinking that can accompany anything meaningful. In these times, we can use our breath to speak calm and focus into our philia. Remember that simply by taking positive actions, you have decided not to take a destructive one. This is a win that should be celebrated! And while this might seem difficult at first, your unconscious-self will slowly learn these new patterns of behavior and assist you more readily in the future.

Breathe messages of calm, using breathing techniques from this book that you have practiced regularly. Don't wait until the moment when you need the technique to send an important message to your unconscious-self to try it for the first time.

Before you take positive action, breathe in a way that will help your philia stay calm. As you take positive action, breathe in a way to remain calm. After you have taken positive action, breathe with a smile, knowing that you have done more than just a simple task. You have worked with your unconscious-self as a team, stronger than ever before. You have avoided destructive behavior, and you have acted positively. In addition to that, you have taught your unconscious-self that you are a person who can think under pressure and take positive action. Never underestimate the power of this victory.

Dealing with Times When You Cannot Act

There are many times when we need to deal with the fact that we simply cannot take action to improve a situation. These are times when we often suffer from rumination and dread. In these times, the unconscious-self continues to ask the conscious-self to think critically about the situation in the hopes that you can solve it on that level. Of course, consciously you might realize that you cannot solve the problem of your loved one being sick or of an impending hurricane, but your unconscious-self, always trying to help you survive and thrive, will continue to feed you dopamine and stress hormones, trying to help you take action. What do we do in times like these?

In these times, what happens all too often is that we become paralyzed with anxiety. There are many things that you can do to improve your life or the lives of others. In many cases, we ignore things that we actually need to do because we are so overwhelmed. This can cause a whole new list of reasons to be stressed.

So how do we deal with paralyzing overwhelm?

BECOMING AWARE   In these times, you are probably very aware of the feelings that you have, but the Awareness Exercise is essential. Take the time to be fully aware of your emotional and autonomic state. Use your sense of internal awareness. Don't make any judgments. Just become aware.

SITTING WITH THE FEELING   The Listening Exercise is ideal for times when you cannot do anything to change the thing that is bothering you. In many cases, we are tormented by things that happened in the past or things that might happen in the future. The Listening Exercise gives us an opportunity to sit with these emotions and safely allow ourselves to be present with them. Remember that your unconscious-self is always trying to help you, and that these emotions are coming from a place of love and are not a sign of anything wrong with you. After practicing the Listening

Exercise, most practitioners feel more at ease with whatever the issue is. Often, practitioners will realize there are things that they can do, but they were so stressed that they couldn't think of them. Most of our suffering comes from our tendency to avoid our emotions. The Listening Exercise is a way to engage them directly, safely, and effectively.

PRACTICING SUPERVENTILATION　While a daily Listening Exercise session is ideal, you might need to interrupt your ruminations and anxieties at a separate time. A purposeful superventilation session might be exactly what you need. Choose any of the protocols from chapter 12, play some pleasant music, and give yourself an opportunity to interrupt the dopamine feedback loop that can often cause us to ruminate and stress over things we cannot do anything about.

APPLYING PRESENCE, TONE, AND TECHNIQUES　It is during times of chronic stress that we often see our breathing patterns become erratic and stress-inducing, which is the worst thing that we can let happen, since we are already in a stressed state. Therefore, check in with your breathing regularly. Are you breathing low into your belly? Are you using your nose? Are you breathing with a steady flow rather than an erratic pace? While these are things that you should be doing anyway, it is extra important to maintain these healthy breathing habits in stressful times.

TAKING ACTION WHERE POSSIBLE　We often ruminate when we have nothing to do. While we shouldn't take actions to distract us from our emotions, doing something meaningful rather than ruminating uselessly is a better use of your time. There are probably things that you should be doing rather than worrying about things you cannot do anything about. Put your philia to good use, maintaining internal awareness and communicating with your unconscious-self with every breath as you go.

Making a Major Change

Maybe you want to make a big change in your life. This can look very different for everyone, but it all comes down to putting yourself in the best state to take positive actions to move yourself toward your goal.

I had a client who was a former career nurse who reached out to me because she dreamed of driving her grandson to the zoo for a fun day. She only had one problem: she was terribly afraid of driving on the highway. When she entered the highway, she would become overwhelmed with anxiety, and she especially disliked driving near semitrucks.

"Here I am, a nurse who has been able to stay cool under intense stress at the hospital, but I can't even drive on the highway," she said, laughing and shaking her head.

When I told her that this was a very common thing and that she was my second client in that month to reach out with the same problem, she couldn't believe it. She thought there was something wrong with her. There wasn't. Her unconscious-self was trying to protect her based on what it believed about the situation of driving on the highway. Our goal was to convince her unconscious-self that this action was something that she was capable of doing without suffering injury or death.

So, what did we do? We had to reteach her unconscious-self, using the process I describe in greater depth in the following section. First, we developed her sense of interoception and improved her rapport with her unconscious-self a great deal before she attempted the drive. We also discovered that she was overcaffeinating herself daily, so we slowly weaned her from regular coffee to decaf. After a few weeks of prep, we moved into the next stage, microexposures.

She really liked the Cadence of Bliss (4,7,8,0), so we decided to make that the technique she would use as she entered the onramp to the highway, and then she used a metronome soundtrack to practice Balanced Breathing or Box Breathing, whichever she found easier in the moment.

First, she simply entered the highway and drove to the first exit. This was a big win. She told me that she was afraid, but she said that knowing that her fear was just her unconscious-self trying to help her made it a little less scary. Over the following days, she repeated this small feat until she felt somewhat comfortable taking this small part of the drive. We kept lengthening the amount of highway she would traverse alone, using her breathing to reassure her unconscious-self, all the while teaching her unconscious-self that she is someone who takes that drive. This process went on for about two months.

Eventually, she made the drive all by herself all the way to the zoo; of course, this meant that she was also making the drive home too. After being diligent and using her breath to speak calm into her philia, she eventually was able to take her grandson to the zoo.

But make no mistake; she wasn't magically made unafraid. She worked for it. When I asked her about the semitrucks, she said that she still never passes them. If she comes upon a slow-driving semitruck, she just stays behind them. I asked her if she wanted to work on passing semitrucks, but with her usual smile and laugh, she quickly said that she was happy with her new normal for now and not quite ready to push any farther.

For this client, she reached her goal, and that was enough. She set a realistic goal, and she took the actions to achieve it. While driving on the highway might not seem like a big thing for some, it changed this client's life and allowed her to take the actions that she wanted to take. There will be limits, but the next section will cover the steps that I recommend for making these kinds of changes.

Teaching in the Way That Humans Learn

We often seek to make overnight changes. This is an example of the conscious-self knowing what the end goal should look like without considering that the unconscious-self will likely need some time to get on board. Our patterns, habits, and personalities are things that the unconscious-self governs. Expecting our unconscious-self to suddenly change because we have a conscious desire to do so is not a realistic strategy for most people. To the best of our unconscious-selves' knowledge, these old habits and patterns have been keeping us alive, safe, and possibly thriving.

You will also have to contend with the fact that your unconscious-self has been putting together a conception of what you are capable of and what you are not capable of. It has also been putting together a conception of the way the world works. These conceptions are difficult to change; I will not lie. However, in my own personal experience, and in the experience of many of my clients, positive change is possible. The unconscious-self is incredibly good at discovering patterns, but it can take some time to let them go. You will have to have a lot of conscious determination, but it is possible to show your unconscious-self a new pattern, one where you can do the thing you have been afraid to do. When clients ask me for help in these areas, my advice is to use the protocol in the following section.

Overcoming Limiting Beliefs and Fear

To demonstrate a method of using the Language of Breath Philosophy to overcome limiting beliefs and fears that often keep us from taking actions to improve our lives, we will use the example of social anxiety. However, the following considerations could apply to nearly anything.

One of the most common things that people ask me about is how to become more comfortable in social situations. They have become convinced that they cannot be comfortable making introductions, making small talk, or speaking to groups of people. They will say that they are introverts, so they are simply not "wired" for being social. Or they will point to how anxious they become, which leaves them unable to think of anything to say. Of course, the list goes on and on, but if you are in this camp, rest assured that you are not alone. If this does not sound like you, you can apply the following method to most other instances where fear and anxiety are getting in the way of you taking the actions that you would like to take in life.

In the case of the introvert who wants to become more outgoing, here is a protocol that you can use.

1. **Lean into the Awareness Exercise so that you can become proficient enough to practice the Advanced Awareness Exercise.** When you practice the Advanced Awareness Exercise, allow yourself to think about an upcoming possibility to be social. Allow yourself to become aware of the subtle (and sometimes not-so-subtle) ways that your unconscious-self reacts to this thought. We will come back to this regularly to gauge progress.

2. **The Listening Exercise can be a powerful tool in cases such as this.** Allow yourself to think about an opportunity that you might have to be social at the beginning of your session and let that be the focus. Using

your sense of internal awareness, focus on the social opportunity and the physical sensations that arise from thinking about it. Then begin the session and allow yourself to be open to listening to what your unconscious-self has to say about it, knowing that it is only trying to help you survive and thrive in your environment and culture. When we listen, we often uncover things that can help us in our journey that we have avoided due to the discomfort that this part of life has been associated with. Really dedicate yourself to listening and understanding.

3. **Affect labeling** is an effective strategy to help remove the scariness from unconscious emotions about something. This means we try to describe in words what we are feeling and why we are feeling it. This is easier to do after the Listening Exercise, but it can be done anytime. Simply by attaching words to the emotions, we can bring them into the conscious space and remove the ambiguity that can make them seem more intimidating and difficult to face.

4. **Develop a regular rapport with your unconscious-self by breathing functionally and using techniques often.** The prep work helps, but you will still need to do the work of doing the thing that brings you so much fear so you can demonstrate to your unconscious-self that you are someone who can do this action and that the world is not as unsafe as you once thought. Use what you now know about breathing calm into your philia all through the day and apply what you know to help you relax enough to take the action that you want to take.

The most common mistake that I see in clients and breathwork enthusiasts is waiting until they are hyperanxious before using their breath to communicate calm to the unconscious. If we wait until we feel incredibly anxious, we have waited for the unconscious-self to scream at us. Have a little consideration for the unconscious-you and speak calm into your philia with every breath so that when moments arise for you to take the actions that you wish to take, you are in the right state. While you will likely feel very anxious in the beginning of your journey, remember that this feeling is only coming from a part of you that is trying to protect you. It is acting out of love, and there is nothing wrong with you. In time, you will train your unconscious-self to see this new experience as normal.

5. **Choose your microexposures and use your breath to remind your unconscious-self that you are safe.** A microexposure is a small exposure to whatever you are afraid to do. While life will not always allow you to choose the times when you are in certain situations, if you can plan for daily microexposures to social situations, this is an excellent way to say to your unconscious-self, "See? I am good at talking to others and being social."

The goal is to pick microexposures that are challenging but easy enough that you will have a good chance at success. We are looking for wins here. If you typically have difficulty making conversation at dinner parties, a good goal would be to try to make small talk in the lunch line or to try to say "hello" to everyone you see in the hallways at work. Or you might simply decide to attempt to have one conversation the next time you are at a dinner party. If you skip these small exposures and go right to inviting twenty people to your house for a dinner party, you have probably put too much on yourself.

Use your breath to remind your unconscious-self that you are having fun and are safe. When I teach this to clients, I like to share the way my wife and I coach each other when we occasionally have to drag each other to events that the other is not excited for. What always happens is that one of us doesn't want to go, but the other does. So, the one who wants to go will remind the other of how much fun we are having and point out how much fun the event is. Before the event is over, we are usually both having a blast (or at least not having as bad a time as one of us thought we would). Good partners put up with their other half and are attentive to their needs; you can put up with your unconscious-self and be attentive too. Just remember that you will need to remind yourself of how much fun you are having, employing your favorite breathing techniques and using functional breathing as you go.

6. **The new normal: a.k.a. better is better!** Reaching a goal is not a single-step process. You will have many steps along the way, and since you are not a machine, you will always have room to grow and improve.

It is important to recognize growth along the way. We often call this the state of "the new normal." Perhaps you once had trouble socializing and your goal is to be a social butterfly. While some people might make that big leap, most of us will need to be patient and make gradual progress. It is important to celebrate your progress.

As you continue to make progress, remember to continue to practice the Awareness Exercise and the Listening Exercise. These practices can help you notice the progress that you have made. However, there is no greater gauge for progress than observing yourself being a little more willing to engage socially, a little more comfortable talking in groups, or maybe even a little excited to attend a social gathering. Every time you take positive action, you are demonstrating to yourself that you are someone who can! Maybe you've not arrived at the status of social king or queen just yet, but better is always better. Look at how far you've come as evidence that you can make positive changes. You are not stuck. Celebrate this journey!

Other Considerations

CO_2 TOLERANCE TRAINING Improving your CO_2 tolerance can be very helpful when it comes to overcoming fear that gets in the way of taking the actions you wish to take. This should be done at times when you are not stressed to avoid exacerbating the feelings of stress. For most people, first thing in the morning and right before bed are optimal times.

SUPERVENTILATION PROTOCOLS While it will likely be impossible to drop to the floor and begin practicing the Interruption Protocol or Sniff Sniff Poo, these protocols are often very helpful right before engaging in a microexposure or a time of full-on challenge. Superventilation can help us stop overthinking, which is common when we are about to engage in an activity that we normally avoid due to fear. Your unconscious-self has kicked up a flurry of emotions and alerts that it is asking you to consciously examine and figure out. But the truth is that your best bet in these situations is to lean more on your personality and sense of humor, things that your unconscious-self is more suited for. It is in these times that we can use superventilation to relax the conscious-self and give the unconscious-self a nudge to do what it does so well. We often refer to this as inducing a state of flow, which is exactly what you want to do rather than trying to manage everything with your conscious thinking. So, do a quality session before you engage your fear; then go into the situation breathing with the tone and presence that you know will keep your philia calm and ready to take positive action, speaking with breathing techniques when you feel the need.

REMEMBER WHERE FEAR COMES FROM   The example of social anxiety is just one example that shows a practical way to move yourself to take actions that you want to take but might be afraid to. Fear is coming from your unconscious-self, and it is only there to try to help you to avoid danger. It is strange to think about self-limiting fears as coming from a place of love, but this is the case. It is important not to resent yourself for this. Not only will it not help you get any closer to taking positive actions, but it is also just one more way to reinforce the belief that you are stuck.

IS IT REALLY FEAR?   Remember that two people can be standing side by side, getting ready to do the same thing, experiencing the same level of autonomic nervous system activation, and while one is anxious, the other is excited. Remember that your unconscious-self is trying to put you into the best state to take positive action. Be willing to interpret your state as something that will help you rather than something that will hinder you. You will certainly need energy to be a social butterfly. You will certainly need alertness to be present in conversations. If you feel that your unconscious-self is activating you for action, in addition to speaking calm and confidence back into your philia with each breath, why not go with it? Why not use that energy to smile and interact with others (or engage in whatever activity that you might have been avoiding due to fear)? You might find that your unconscious-self is giving you exactly the state that you need, and all you need to do is work with it rather than against it. The next time you feel anxious, consider that this might be excitement instead.

The Never-Ending Communication

There is no way to predict the situations or the struggles that you will face in your lifetime, but with this new understanding of what you are and how you interact within yourself, you can face any obstacle as the singular organism that you are, a conscious and unconscious team that is you. Life is an event that will not end until you die. Let every breath be an opportunity to create a positive relationship within yourself, and may every action you take lead you to a better life.

CONCLUSION

THE FORWARD-FACING PHILIA

You are not a machine. You are not a tree. You are a human, an incredible relationship of trillions of cells working together to take positive actions to survive and thrive on planet Earth. At every moment, at all times, there is no part of you that isn't you, and how you interact with yourself will determine the health of this incredible team, which is you. What actions will you take now that you have learned to communicate within yourself? What new heights will you reach? Who will you reach out to?

Let today be the dawn of a new era in your life—one of connection and self-compassion, knowing that there is nothing that your team cannot do. This should also be a time when you examine how you are treating yourself. Are you treating yourself like a machine? Or are you treating yourself like a living, breathing, feeling creature who is biologically driven to take action?

With our new understanding of what we are and how we can play an active role within ourselves, we can approach future situations with even more confidence, knowing that this team that we all carry within us can work together to accomplish amazing things. Take care of your philia. Take care of yourself.

AFTERWORD

RICHARD BOSTOCK

It brings me great joy to pen a few words to conclude this wonderful book written by my brother in breath, Jesse. I feel that Jesse and I are cut from the same cloth in that when we come across something that lights us up, it instantly becomes an obsession to understand it completely. When it comes to the ancient and yet ever-evolving art of using breath with purpose and intention, understanding it completely is certainly a daunting prospect that will perhaps take more than a lifetime to truly master. I'm sure I can speak for Jesse when I say that we will both forever humbly be students of the breath.

What Jesse has accomplished with this book is to provide a unique framework of understanding and implementing breathwork, not just as a collection of techniques, but as a philosophy to be explored. This is what I appreciate most about Jesse and his teaching philosophy. Too many times we see teachers or schools silo themselves within a selected set of techniques and beliefs of what the breath can do, rather than see it as ever-evolving dynamic interplay of all aspects of the human experience. If this seems confusing to you, I'd like to share a personal story of when the penny dropped for me.

While I was on retreat with one of my teachers, he sent me away with a task of practicing (and hopefully perfecting) a certain breathwork technique. After several days of constant practice, I felt as though I had the technique mastered, and I went to him to demonstrate all my good work. After seeing that I was proficient in the technique, he then told me to go away and start practicing the exact opposite of what I had just spent days perfecting. Chuckling at my puzzled look, he explained that mastery of breathwork is not about perfecting a technique; it's about experiencing every aspect of breath so that you can cultivate your own felt-sense relationship with it, embodying its own expression of how it can manifest within you.

Of course, certain aspects of breathwork can be and should be very mechanical, such as understanding the optimal muscular mechanics that best support us, such as diaphragmatic breathing at rest or strengthening primary and accessory breathing muscles for increased athletic performance. The world now understands the importance of nasal breathing and how CO_2 tolerance training can bring great benefit. Scientific research is continuing to quantify how different techniques, specific ratios, and various aspects of breath affect our physiology. But the possibilities of what the breath can bring aren't always linear, quantifiable, or mechanical. Breathwork is not a straight line; it is a wiggle. It is the inspirational point where science meets art. Where understanding becomes feeling. Where the objective and rational dissolves into the esoteric and mysterious. To quote French composer Claude Debussy, "Music is the space between the notes."

As Jesse so eloquently encapsulates in his book, we are moving toward a new paradigm of understanding the human experience. One that considers the human being as a complex system of conscious and unconscious thought, emotion, subtle energy, and physicality interacting within an environment. Each aspect of this universal intelligence that we call "human" is constantly communicating and informing the other and cannot be separated. So, the question now is, how can the breath serve you?

The uniqueness of the breath is that it acts as a bridge across every aspect of self. Connection with your breath can down-regulate stress and anxiety, improve sleep, increase creativity, bring greater clarity of thought and insight, aid in the healing of physical illness and disease, provide greater connection to loved ones, liberate you from emotional trauma, and even provide a glimpse into the nonphysical realms of existence. For me, above all, the breath has taken me by the hand and has guided me on the greatest adventure that I believe anyone can embark on: the adventure to answer the question, "Who am I really?"

Congratulations to Jesse for creating this ode to the breath that I am certain will serve many people. The breath has so much to offer to us all, and it is my greatest wish that the readers of this book let the breath guide them toward endless possibility.

HEALTH CONSIDERATIONS

Superventilation and Circular Breathing Safety Considerations

Passing out   When we practice any kind of breathwork that lowers CO_2 levels, we also increase the likelihood of passing out. A big reduction in CO_2 can cause vasoconstriction in blood vessels while reducing the ability of the brain to absorb oxygen due to the Bohr effect. This is why any use of superventilation should be done lying down or in a seated position on the floor. Never practice superventilation or any circular breathing technique in water, while driving, or in any situation where losing consciousness could cause you to fall, drown, or lose control of machinery.

Tetany   This is a common issue when practicing superventilation techniques. It involves involuntary muscle contractions due to overly stimulated peripheral nerves due to the imbalance in electrolytes that can accompany a shift in blood pH, usually a temporary dip in blood levels of calcium. While this is normally not dangerous, in extreme cases a brief period of very low calcium levels (hypocalcemia) can result in seizures. In the Language of Breath Philosophy, we take measures to avoid this, so practicing the techniques in this book is much safer than most other forms of superventilation out there. However, it is important to be aware of this. Returning to normal breathing will allow the blood pH to normalize, mitigating the symptoms very quickly.

Health Contraindications for Superventilation and the Listening Exercise

Even if you do not suffer from one of the conditions on this list, check with your doctor to make sure that you are healthy enough to practice the superventilation breathwork techniques described in this book.

Epilepsy   Superventilation should be avoided by those who suffer from epilepsy. The low levels of CO_2 in the blood can cause a condition called hypocalcemia. This is a brief state of low calcium in the blood that can lead to a seizure.

Uncontrolled high blood pressure   Superventilation can induce a strong temporary stressed state. This, combined with low CO_2 in the blood, can lead to constriction of blood vessels and a temporary increase in blood pressure that can be dangerous if you already have high blood pressure. See your health care practitioner to find out more about your blood pressure and whether superventilation is right for you.

Recent heart attack or stroke   Since vasoconstriction can occur when practicing superventilation, check with your doctor to ensure you have recovered enough to practice superventilation.

Pregnancy and nursing   Because superventilation can induce a temporary stressed state, it is important to avoid doing this style of breathwork while pregnant or nursing. Heightened levels of stress may impact your baby, so it is best to be on the safe side and wait until you are no longer pregnant or nursing.

Asthma   While the Language of Breath protocols will mitigate this risk factor significantly because we will only breathe through the nose to a balanced cadence, it is still a good idea to keep your inhaler handy. In cases of dry air or air with dust or pollen floating around, increased airflow can lead to inflammation of the upper airways.

Psychiatric conditions   Individuals who suffer from bipolar disorder, schizophrenia, personality disorders, or any dramatic breathwork requiring hospitalization should only use this style of breathwork in the presence of a highly qualified breathworker and under the supervision of a therapist.

ACKNOWLEDGMENTS

To my wife, Nicole. Thank you for supporting me and never letting me give up on my passion for helping others through breath. It is no exaggeration to say that I would not be the man I am today without you.

I want to thank my friend Martin McPhilimey for your friendship and your willingness to read my work and offer such great feedback. I am grateful to have met you at the perfect time. For anyone who would like to learn more from Martin, please visit www.performancethroughhealth.com.

Thank you, Tom Granger, for your feedback and for teaching me about Resonance Frequency Breathing. For anyone who would like to learn more from Tom, please visit him at www.AriaBreath.com.

Thank you, Dr. Otto Muzik. You have been a mentor and a friend over the years, and I have learned so much from you. Thank you for your honest and constructive criticisms, your deep lessons, and your good sense of humor. My breathwork practice would not be what it is today without our regular conversations.

To all of the great teachers and influences I have had over the years, I thank you! For some, you have taught me directly, and for others, you have influenced me indirectly. I am grateful either way. Thank you, Kasper van der Meulen, Paul Hughes, Wim Hof, Brian Mackenzie, Patrick Mckeown, Michaël Bijker, Jim Leonard, Richard Bostock, and Niraj Naik. Thank you for your voice and for teaching me more than you might ever know.

NOTES

Introduction

1 Centers for Disease Control and Prevention, "Type 2 Diabetes," December 16, 2021, www.cdc.gov/diabetes/basics/type2.html#:~:text=Healthy%20eating%20is%20 your%20recipe,them%20have%20type%202%20diabetes.

2 Centers for Disease Control and Prevention, "Prediabetes—Your Chance to Prevent Type 2 Diabetes," December 21, 2021, www.cdc.gov/diabetes/basics/prediabetes.html.

3 Jung Ha Park, Ji Hyun Moon, Hyeon Ju Kim, Mi Hee Kong, and Yun Hwan Oh, "Sedentary Lifestyle: Overview of Updated Evidence of Potential Health Risks," *Korean Journal of Family Medicine* 41, no. 6 (2020): 365–73, https://doi.org/10.4082/kjfm.20.0165.

4 Jane E. Ferrie, Meena Kumari, Paula Salo, Archana Singh-Manoux, and Mika Kivimäki, "Sleep Epidemiology—A Rapidly Growing Field," *International Journal of Epidemiology* 40, no. 6 (2011): 1431–37, https://doi.org/10.1093/ije/dyr203.

5 Harvard Health, "GERD: Heartburn and More," March 1, 2008, www.health.harvard .edu/staying-healthy/gerd-heartburn-and-more.

6 Borwin Bandelow and Sophie Michaelis, "Epidemiology of Anxiety Disorders in the 21st Century," *Dialogues in Clinical Neuroscience* 17, no. 3 (2015): 327–35, https://doi.org /10.31887/dcns.2015.17.3/bbandelow.

7 Centers for Disease Control and Prevention, "Life Expectancy in the U.S. Dropped for the Second Year in a Row in 2021," August 31, 2022, www.cdc.gov/nchs/pressroom /nchs_press_releases/2022/20220831.htm.

8 Aditi Nerurkar, Asaf Bitton, Roger B. Davis, Russell S. Phillips, and Gloria Yeh, "When Physicians Counsel about Stress: Results of a National Study," *JAMA Internal Medicine* 173, no. 1 (2013): 76, https://doi.org/10.1001/2013.jamainternmed.480.

9 Alicia E. Meuret, Thomas Ritz, Frank H. Wilhelm, and Walton T. Roth, "Voluntary Hyperventilation in the Treatment of Panic Disorder—Functions of Hyperventilation, Their Implications for Breathing Training, and Recommendations for Standardization," *Clinical Psychology Review* 25, no. 3 (2005): 285–306, https://doi .org/10.1016/j.cpr.2005.01.002.

10 Leon Chaitow, Dinah Bradley, Christopher Gilbert, Jim Bartley, and David Peters, *Recognizing and Treating Breathing Disorders: A Multidisciplinary Approach* (Edinburgh: Churchill Livingstone/Elsevier, 2018).

1. Misconceptions Lead to Disconnections

1   David Young, "*Mens Sana in Corpore Sano?* Body and Mind in Ancient Greece," *International Journal of the History of Sport* 22, no. 1 (2005): 22–41, https://doi.org/10.1080/0952336 052000314638.

2   Gert-Jan Lokhorst, "Descartes and the Pineal Gland," Stanford Encyclopedia of Philosophy, September 18, 2013, https://plato.stanford.edu/entries/pineal-gland.

3   Emma Young, "Lifting the Lid on the Unconscious," *New Scientist,* July 26, 2018, www.newscientist.com/article/mg23931880-400-lifting-the-lid-on-the-unconscious.

4   Drew Westen, "The Scientific Status of Unconscious Processes: Is Freud Really Dead?" *Journal of the American Psychoanalytic Association* 47, no. 4 (1999): 1061–1106, https://doi.org/10.1177/00030651990470040404; Timothy D. Wilson, *Strangers to Ourselves: Discovering the Adaptive Unconscious* (Cambridge, MA: Belknap, 2004).

5   Emily Kwong and Pragya Agarwal, "Understanding Unconscious Bias," NPR, July 15, 2020, www.npr.org/2020/07/14/891140598/understanding-unconscious-bias.

6   Wilson, *Strangers to Ourselves.*

7   Wilson, *Strangers to Ourselves.*

2. Action Is the Strategy

1   Cleveland Clinic, "Cortisol," December 10, 2021, https://my.clevelandclinic.org/health /articles/22187-cortisol.

2   Raj Chovatiya and Ruslan Medzhitov, "Stress, Inflammation, and Defense of Homeostasis," *Molecular Cell* 54, no. 2 (2014): 281–88, https://doi.org/10.1016/j.molcel.2014.03.030.

3   Robyn R. M. Gershon, Briana Barocas, Allison N. Canton, Xianbin Li, and David Vlahov, "Mental, Physical, and Behavioral Outcomes Associated with Perceived Work Stress in Police Officers," *Criminal Justice and Behavior* 36, no. 3 (2008): 275–89, https://doi.org/10.1177/0093854808330015; Arne Nieuwenhuys, Geert J. P. Savelsbergh, and Raôul R. D. Oudejans, "Persistence of Threat-Induced Errors in Police Officers' Shooting Decisions," *Applied Ergonomics* 48 (2015): 263–72, https://doi.org/10.1016/j .apergo.2014.12.006; Mathias Luethi, "Stress Effects on Working Memory, Explicit Memory, and Implicit Memory for Neutral and Emotional Stimuli in Healthy Men," *Frontiers in Behavioral Neuroscience* 2 (2009), https://doi.org/10.3389/neuro.08.005.2008; Milena Girotti, Samantha M. Adler, Sarah E. Bulin, Elizabeth A. Fucich, Denisse

Paredes, and David A. Morilak, "Prefrontal Cortex Executive Processes Affected by Stress in Health and Disease," *Progress in Neuro-Psychopharmacology and Biological Psychiatry* 85 (2018): 161–79, https://doi.org/10.1016/j.pnpbp.2017.07.004.

7. Learning Breath Mechanics

1 Yuka Shimozawa, Toshiyuki Kurihara, Yuki Kusagawa, Miyuki Hori, Shun Numasawa, Takashi Sugiyama, Takahiro Tanaka, et al., "Point Prevalence of the Biomechanical Dimension of Dysfunctional Breathing Patterns Among Competitive Athletes," *Journal of Strength and Conditioning Research,* May 24, 2022, https://doi.org/10.1519/jsc.0000000000004253.

2 SeYoon Kim, JuHyeon Jung, and NanSoo Kim, "The Effects of McKenzie Exercise on Forward Head Posture and Respiratory Function," *Journal of Korean Physical Therapy* 31, no. 6 (December 30, 2019): 351–57, https://doi.org/10.18857/jkpt.2019.31.6.351.

3 Mitch Lomax, Ian Grant, and Jo Corbett, "Inspiratory Muscle Warm-up and Inspiratory Muscle Training: Separate and Combined Effects on Intermittent Running to Exhaustion," *Journal of Sports Sciences* 29, no. 6 (March 2011): 563–69, https://doi.org/10.1080/02640414.2010.543911.

9. Build a Vocabulary for Every Occasion

1 Eddie Weitzberg and Jon O. N. Lundberg, "Humming Greatly Increases Nasal Nitric Oxide," *American Journal of Respiratory and Critical Care Medicine* 166, no. 2 (July 15, 2002): 144–45, https://doi.org/10.1164/rccm.200202-138bc.

2 Paul M. Lehrer, Evgeny Vaschillo, and Bronya Vaschillo, "Resonant Frequency Biofeedback Training to Increase Cardiac Variability: Rationale and Manual for Training," *Applied Psychophysiology and Biofeedback* 25, no. 3 (September 2000): 177–91, https://doi.org/10.1023/a:1009554825745.

3 Patrick R. Steffen, Tara Austin, Andrea DeBarros, and Tracy Brown, "The Impact of Resonance Frequency Breathing on Measures of Heart Rate Variability, Blood Pressure, and Mood," *Frontiers in Public Health* 5 (August 25, 2017), https://doi.org/10.3389/fpubh.2017.00222.

4 Stephen W. Porges, *Polyvagal Safety: Attachment, Communication, Self-Regulation* (New York: W. W. Norton, 2021).

10. Love Your Nose

1 Christopher Gilbert, "Interaction of Psychological and Emotional Variables with Breathing Dysfunction," in *Recognizing and Treating Breathing Disorders: A Multidisciplinary*

Approach, ed. Leon Chaitow, Dinah Bradley, and Christopher Gilbert (Edinburgh, UK: Churchill Livingstone/Elsevier, 2018), 79–91.

2 J. O. N. Lundberg, G. Settergren, S. Gelinder, J. M. Lundberg, K. Alving, and E. Weitzberg, "Inhalation of Nasally Derived Nitric Oxide Modulates Pulmonary Function in Humans," *Acta Physiologica Scandinavica* 158, no. 4 (1996): 343–47, https://doi.org/10.1046/j.1365-201x.1996.557321000.x.

3 M. Antosova, D. Mokra, L. Pepucha, J. Plevkova, T. Buday, M. Sterusky, and A. Bencova, "Physiology of Nitric Oxide in the Respiratory System," *Physiological Research* 66, Suppl. 2 (2017): S159–72, https://doi.org/10.33549/physiolres.933673.

4 Sophie Svensson, Anna Carin Olin, and Johan Hellgren, "Increased Net Water Loss by Oral Compared to Nasal Expiration in Healthy Subjects," *Rhinology* 44, no. 1 (March 2006): 74–7. https://pubmed.ncbi.nlm.nih.gov/16550955/.

5 K. P. Strohl, J. L. Arnold, M. J. Decker, P. L. Hoekje, and E. R. McFadden, "Nasal Flow-Resistive Responses to Challenge with Cold Dry Air," *Journal of Applied Physiology* 72, no. 4 (1992): 1243–46, https://doi.org/10.1152/jappl.1992.72.4.1243.

11. Team Building

1 Donald F. Klein, "False Suffocation Alarms, Spontaneous Panics, and Related Conditions," *Archives of General Psychiatry* 50, no. 4 (1993): 306, https://doi.org/10.1001/archpsyc.1993.01820160076009; George Savulich, Frank H. Hezemans, Sophia van Ghesel Grothe, Jessica Dafflon, Norah Schulten, Annette B. Brühl, Barbara J. Sahakian, and Trevor W. Robbins, "Acute Anxiety and Autonomic Arousal Induced by CO_2 Inhalation Impairs Prefrontal Executive Functions in Healthy Humans," *Translational Psychiatry* 9, no. 1 (2019), https://doi.org/10.1038/s41398-019-0634-z.

2 Henry D. Covelli, J. Waylon Black, Michael S. Olsen, and Jerome F. Beekman, "Respiratory Failure Precipitated by High Carbohydrate Loads," *Annals of Internal Medicine* 95, no. 5 (November 1, 1981): 579, https://doi.org/10.7326/0003-4819-95-5-579.

3 David Beales, "Breath, Buffers and Performance," *Functional Sports Nutrition,* March–April 2014: 8–10, www.equinebreathing.com/uploads/Files/65_breath_buffers_performance_d_beales.pdf; Johnny E. Brian, "Carbon Dioxide and the Cerebral Circulation," *Anesthesiology* 88, no. 5 (May 1, 1998): 1365–86, https://doi.org/10.1097/00000542-199805000-00029.

12. Superventilation, Circular Breathing, Hypocapnia, and Bliss

1 Joseph P. Rhinewine and Oliver J. Williams, "Holotropic Breathwork: The Potential Role of a Prolonged, Voluntary Hyperventilation Procedure as an Adjunct to Psychotherapy,"

Journal of Alternative and Complementary Medicine 13, no. 7 (November 7, 2007): 771–76, https://doi.org/10.1089/acm.2006.6203.

2 H. Scholz, H.-J. Schurek, K.-U. Eckardt, and C. Bauer, "Role of Erythropoietin in Adaptation to Hypoxia," *Experientia* 46, no. 11–12 (December 1, 1990): 1197–1201, https://doi.org/10.1007/bf01936936.

3 Rhinewine and Williams, "Holotropic Breathwork."

13. Connect to Emotions

1 Lauri Nummenmaa, Enrico Glerean, Riitta Hari, and Jari K. Hietanen, "Bodily Maps of Emotions," *Proceedings of the National Academy of Sciences* 111, no. 2 (December 30, 2013): 646–51, https://doi.org/10.1073/pnas.1321664111; Sahib S. Khalsa, Ralph Adolphs, Oliver G. Cameron, Hugo D. Critchley, Paul W. Davenport, Justin S. Feinstein, Jamie D. Feusner, et al., "Interoception and Mental Health: A Roadmap," *Biological Psychiatry: Cognitive Neuroscience and Neuroimaging* 3, no. 6 (June 2018): 501–13, https://doi.org/10.1016/j.bpsc.2017.12.004.

2 Antoine Bechara, "The Role of Emotion in Decision-Making: Evidence from Neurological Patients with Orbitofrontal Damage," *Brain and Cognition* 55, no. 1 (January 29, 2004): 30–40, https://doi.org/10.1016/j.bandc.2003.04.001.

3 Timothy D. Wilson, *Strangers to Ourselves: Discovering the Adaptive Unconscious* (Cambridge, MA: Belknap, 2004).

4 Nummenmaa et al., "Bodily Maps of Emotions."

5 Cynthia J. Price, and Helen Y. Weng, "Facilitating Adaptive Emotion Processing and Somatic Reappraisal via Sustained Mindful Interoceptive Attention," *Frontiers in Psychology* 12 (September 8, 2021), https://doi.org/10.3389/fpsyg.2021.578827.

6 Regina C. Lapate, Bas Rokers, Tianyi Li, and Richard J. Davidson, "Nonconscious Emotional Activation Colors First Impressions," *Psychological Science* 25, no. 2 (December 6, 2013): 349–57, https://doi.org/10.1177/0956797613503175.

7 Price and Weng, "Facilitating Adaptive Emotion Processing."

14. Use the Language of Breath to Take Positive Actions

1 Sylvain Laborde, Thomas Hosang, Emma Mosley, and Fabrice Dosseville, "Influence of a 30-Day Slow-Paced Breathing Intervention Compared to Social Media Use on Subjective Sleep Quality and Cardiac Vagal Activity," *Journal of Clinical Medicine* 8, no. 2 (February 6, 2019): 193, https://doi.org/10.3390/jcm8020193.

2 Milena Girotti, Samantha M. Adler, Sarah E. Bulin, Elizabeth A. Fucich, Denisse Paredes, and David A. Morilak, "Prefrontal Cortex Executive Processes Affected by Stress in Health and Disease," *Progress in Neuro-Psychopharmacology and Biological Psychiatry* 85 (2018): 161–79, https://doi.org/10.1016/j.pnpbp.2017.07.004.

BIBLIOGRAPHY

Antosova, M., D. Mokra, L. Pepucha, J. Plevkova, T. Buday, M. Sterusky, and A. Bencova. "Physiology of Nitric Oxide in the Respiratory System." *Physiological Research* 66, Suppl. 2 (2017): S159–72. https://doi.org/10.33549/physiolres.933673.

Bandelow, Borwin, and Sophie Michaelis. "Epidemiology of Anxiety Disorders in the 21st Century." *Dialogues in Clinical Neuroscience* 17, no. 3 (2015): 327–35. https://doi.org/10.31887/dcns.2015.17.3/bbandelow.

Beales, David. "Breath, Buffers and Performance." *Functional Sports Nutrition,* March–April 2014: 8–10. www.equinebreathing.com/uploads/Files/65_breath_buffers_performance_d_beales.pdf.

Bechara, Antoine. "The Role of Emotion in Decision-Making: Evidence from Neurological Patients with Orbitofrontal Damage." *Brain and Cognition* 55, no. 1 (January 29, 2004): 30–40. https://doi.org/10.1016/j.bandc.2003.04.001.

Brian, Johnny E. "Carbon Dioxide and the Cerebral Circulation." *Anesthesiology* 88, no. 5 (May 1, 1998): 1365–86. https://doi.org/10.1097/00000542-199805000-00029.

Burke, Kenneth. *The Philosophy of Literary Form: Studies in Symbolic Action.* Baton Rouge, LA: Louisiana State University Press, 1941.

Centers for Disease Control and Prevention. "Life Expectancy in the U.S. Dropped for the Second Year in a Row in 2021." August 31, 2022. www.cdc.gov/nchs/pressroom/nchs_press_releases/2022/20220831.htm.

Centers for Disease Control and Prevention. "Prediabetes—Your Chance to Prevent Type 2 Diabetes." December 21, 2021. www.cdc.gov/diabetes/basics/prediabetes.html.

Centers for Disease Control and Prevention. "Type 2 Diabetes." December 16, 2021. www.cdc.gov/diabetes/basics/type2.html.

Chaitow, Leon, Dinah Bradley, Christopher Gilbert, Jim Bartley, and David Peters. *Recognizing and Treating Breathing Disorders: A Multidisciplinary Approach.* Edinburgh: Churchill Livingstone/Elsevier, 2018.

Chovatiya, Raj, and Ruslan Medzhitov. "Stress, Inflammation, and Defense of Homeostasis." *Molecular Cell* 54, no. 2 (2014): 281–88. https://doi.org/10.1016/j.molcel.2014.03.030.

Cleveland Clinic. "Cortisol." December 10, 2021. https://my.clevelandclinic.org/health/articles/22187-cortisol.

Covelli, Henry D., J. Waylon Black, Michael S. Olsen, and Jerome F. Beekman. "Respiratory Failure Precipitated by High Carbohydrate Loads." *Annals of Internal Medicine* 95, no. 5 (November 1, 1981): 579. https://doi.org/10.7326/0003-4819-95-5-579.

Ferrie, Jane E., Meena Kumari, Paula Salo, Archana Singh-Manoux, and Mika Kivimäki. "Sleep Epidemiology—A Rapidly Growing Field." *International Journal of Epidemiology* 40, no. 6 (2011): 1431–37. https://doi.org/10.1093/ije/dyr203.

Gershon, Robyn R. M., Briana Barocas, Allison N. Canton, Xianbin Li, and David Vlahov. "Mental, Physical, and Behavioral Outcomes Associated with Perceived Work Stress in Police Officers." *Criminal Justice and Behavior* 36, no. 3 (2009): 275–89. https://doi.org/10.1177/0093854808330015.

Gilbert, Christopher. "Interaction of Psychological and Emotional Variables with Breathing Dysfunction." In *Recognizing and Treating Breathing Disorders: A Multidisciplinary Approach,* edited by Leon Chaitow, Dinah Bradley, and Christopher Gilbert, 79–91. Edinburgh, UK: Churchill Livingstone/Elsevier, 2018.

Girotti, Milena, Samantha M. Adler, Sarah E. Bulin, Elizabeth A. Fucich, Denisse Paredes, and David A. Morilak. "Prefrontal Cortex Executive Processes Affected by Stress in Health and Disease." *Progress in Neuro-Psychopharmacology and Biological Psychiatry* 85 (2018): 161–79. https://doi.org/10.1016/j.pnpbp.2017.07.004.

Harvard Health. "GERD: Heartburn and More." March 1, 2008. www.health.harvard.edu /staying-healthy/gerd-heartburn-and-more.

Khalsa, Sahib S., Ralph Adolphs, Oliver G. Cameron, Hugo D. Critchley, Paul W. Davenport, Justin S. Feinstein, Jamie D. Feusner, Sarah N. Garfinkel, Richard D. Lane, Wolf E. Mehling, et al. "Interoception and Mental Health: A Roadmap." *Biological Psychiatry: Cognitive Neuroscience and Neuroimaging* 3, no. 6 (June 2018): 501–13. https://doi.org /10.1016/j.bpsc.2017.12.004.

Kim, SeYoon, JuHyeon Jung, and NanSoo Kim. "The Effects of McKenzie Exercise on Forward Head Posture and Respiratory Function." *Journal of Korean Physical Therapy* 31, no. 6 (December 30, 2019): 351–57. https://doi.org/10.18857/jkpt.2019.31.6.351.

Klein, Donald F. "False Suffocation Alarms, Spontaneous Panics, and Related Conditions." *Archives of General Psychiatry* 50, no. 4 (1993): 306. https://doi.org/10.1001/archpsyc .1993.01820160076009.

Kwong, Emily, and Pragya Agarwal. "Understanding Unconscious Bias." NPR. July 15, 2020. www.npr.org/2020/07/14/891140598/understanding-unconscious-bias.

Laborde, Sylvain, Thomas Hosang, Emma Mosley, and Fabrice Dosseville. "Influence of a 30-Day Slow-Paced Breathing Intervention Compared to Social Media Use on Subjective Sleep Quality and Cardiac Vagal Activity." *Journal of Clinical Medicine* 8, no. 2 (February 6, 2019): 193. https://doi.org/10.3390/jcm8020193.

Lapate, Regina C., Bas Rokers, Tianyi Li, and Richard J. Davidson. "Nonconscious Emotional Activation Colors First Impressions." *Psychological Science* 25, no. 2 (December 6, 2013): 349–57. https://doi.org/10.1177/0956797613503175.

Lehrer, Paul M., Evgeny Vaschillo, and Bronya Vaschillo. "Resonant Frequency Biofeedback Training to Increase Cardiac Variability: Rationale and Manual for Training." *Applied Psychophysiology and Biofeedback* 25, no. 3 (September 2000): 177–91. https://doi.org/10.1023/a:1009554825745.

Lokhorst, Gert-Jan. "Descartes and the Pineal Gland." Stanford Encyclopedia of Philosophy. September 18, 2013. https://plato.stanford.edu/entries/pineal-gland.

Lomax, Mitch, Ian Grant, and Jo Corbett. "Inspiratory Muscle Warm-up and Inspiratory Muscle Training: Separate and Combined Effects on Intermittent Running to Exhaustion." *Journal of Sports Sciences* 29, no. 6 (March 2011): 563–69. https://doi.org/10.1080/02640414.2010.543911.

Luethi, Mathias. "Stress Effects on Working Memory, Explicit Memory, and Implicit Memory for Neutral and Emotional Stimuli in Healthy Men." *Frontiers in Behavioral Neuroscience* 2 (2009). https://doi.org/10.3389/neuro.08.005.2008.

Lundberg, J. O. N., G. Settergren, S. Gelinder, J. M. Lundberg, K. Alving, and E. Weitzberg. "Inhalation of Nasally Derived Nitric Oxide Modulates Pulmonary Function in Humans." *Acta Physiologica Scandinavica* 158, no. 4 (1996): 343–47. https://doi.org/10.1046/j.1365-201x.1996.557321000.x.

Meuret, Alicia E., Thomas Ritz, Frank H. Wilhelm, and Walton T. Roth. "Voluntary Hyperventilation in the Treatment of Panic Disorder—Functions of Hyperventilation, Their Implications for Breathing Training, and Recommendations for Standardization." *Clinical Psychology Review* 25, no. 3 (2005): 285–306. https://doi.org/10.1016/j.cpr.2005.01.002.

Nerurkar, Aditi, Asaf Bitton, Roger B. Davis, Russell S. Phillips, and Gloria Yeh. "When Physicians Counsel about Stress: Results of a National Study." *JAMA Internal Medicine* 173, no. 1 (2013): 76. https://doi.org/10.1001/2013.jamainternmed.480.

Nieuwenhuys, Arne, Geert J. P. Savelsbergh, and Raôul R. D. Oudejans. "Persistence of Threat-Induced Errors in Police Officers' Shooting Decisions." *Applied Ergonomics* 48 (2015): 263–72. https://doi.org/10.1016/j.apergo.2014.12.006.

Nummenmaa, Lauri, Enrico Glerean, Riitta Hari, and Jari K. Hietanen. "Bodily Maps of Emotions." *Proceedings of the National Academy of Sciences* 111, no. 2 (December 30, 2013): 646–51. https://doi.org/10.1073/pnas.1321664111.

Park, Jung Ha, Ji Hyun Moon, Hyeon Ju Kim, Mi Hee Kong, and Yun Hwan Oh. "Sedentary Lifestyle: Overview of Updated Evidence of Potential Health Risks." *Korean Journal of Family Medicine* 41, no. 6 (2020): 365–73. https://doi.org/10.4082/kjfm.20.0165.

Porges, Stephen W. *Polyvagal Safety: Attachment, Communication, Self-Regulation.* New York: W. W. Norton, 2021.

Price, Cynthia J., and Helen Y. Weng. "Facilitating Adaptive Emotion Processing and Somatic Reappraisal via Sustained Mindful Interoceptive Attention." *Frontiers in Psychology* 12 (September 8, 2021). https://doi.org/10.3389/fpsyg.2021.578827.

Rhinewine, Joseph P., and Oliver J. Williams. "Holotropic Breathwork: The Potential Role of a Prolonged, Voluntary Hyperventilation Procedure as an Adjunct to Psychotherapy."

Journal of Alternative and Complementary Medicine 13, no. 7 (November 7, 2007): 771–76. https://doi.org/10.1089/acm.2006.6203.

Savulich, George, Frank H. Hezemans, Sophia van Ghesel Grothe, Jessica Dafflon, Norah Schulten, Annette B. Brühl, Barbara J. Sahakian, and Trevor W. Robbins. "Acute Anxiety and Autonomic Arousal Induced by CO_2 Inhalation Impairs Prefrontal Executive Functions in Healthy Humans." *Translational Psychiatry* 9, no. 1 (2019). https://doi.org/10.1038/s41398-019-0634-z.

Scholz, H., H.-J. Schurek, K.-U. Eckardt, and C. Bauer. "Role of Erythropoietin in Adaptation to Hypoxia." *Experientia* 46, no. 11–12 (December 1, 1990): 1197–1201. https://doi.org/10.1007/bf01936936.

Shimozawa, Yuka, Toshiyuki Kurihara, Yuki Kusagawa, Miyuki Hori, Shun Numasawa, Takashi Sugiyama, Takahiro Tanaka, Tadashi Suga, Ryoko S. Terada, Tadao Isaka, and Masafumi Terada. "Point Prevalence of the Biomechanical Dimension of Dysfunctional Breathing Patterns Among Competitive Athletes." *Journal of Strength and Conditioning Research* (May 24, 2022), https://doi.org/10.1519/jsc.0000000000004253.

Steffen, Patrick R., Tara Austin, Andrea DeBarros, and Tracy Brown. "The Impact of Resonance Frequency Breathing on Measures of Heart Rate Variability, Blood Pressure, and Mood." *Frontiers in Public Health* 5 (August 25, 2017). https://doi.org/10.3389/fpubh.2017.00222.

Strohl, K. P., J. L. Arnold, M. J. Decker, P. L. Hoekje, and E. R. McFadden. "Nasal Flow-Resistive Responses to Challenge with Cold Dry Air." *Journal of Applied Physiology* 72, no. 4 (1992): 1243–46. https://doi.org/10.1152/jappl.1992.72.4.1243.

Svensson, Sophie, Anna Carin Olin, and Johan Hellgren. "Increased Net Water Loss by Oral Compared to Nasal Expiration in Healthy Subjects." *Rhinology* 44, no. 1 (March 2006).

Weitzberg, Eddie, and Jon O. N. Lundberg. "Humming Greatly Increases Nasal Nitric Oxide." *American Journal of Respiratory and Critical Care Medicine* 166, no. 2 (July 15, 2002): 144–45. https://doi.org/10.1164/rccm.200202-138bc.

Westen, Drew. "The Scientific Status of Unconscious Processes: Is Freud Really Dead?" *Journal of the American Psychoanalytic Association* 47, no. 4 (1999): 1061–1106. https://doi.org/10.1177/00030651990470040.

Wilson, Timothy D. *Strangers to Ourselves: Discovering the Adaptive Unconscious.* Cambridge, MA: Belknap, 2004.

Young, David. "*Mens Sana in Corpore Sano?* Body and Mind in Ancient Greece." *International Journal of the History of Sport* 22, no. 1 (2005): 22–41. https://doi.org/10.1080/0952336052000314638.

Young, Emma. "Lifting the Lid on the Unconscious." *New Scientist.* July 26, 2018. www.newscientist.com/article/mg23931880-400-lifting-the-lid-on-the-unconscious.

INDEX

V

vagus nerve, 95
Vaschillo, Evgeny, 99
Viagra advertisements, 24
vocabulary, 89
  apneas, 93, 109
  Balanced Breathing, 98–100
  becoming an attentive partner, 91
  breathing notation, 92–93
  conversation within us, 89–90
  creating phrases, 109
  forcing conversations, 106–107
  guiding conversations, 108–109
  knowing your role, 91–92
  "Let's Calm Down.", 53–55, 95–97
  "Let's Feel Good and Energize."
    (Peaceful Apneas), 106
  "Let's Feel Good!" (Cadence of Bliss), 105
  "Let's Get Excited!", 97
  "Let's Slow Down and Relax.", 104–105
  "Let's Stay Focused, Relaxed, and
    Centered." (Box Breathing),
    100–102
  need to change paradigm, 94
  practicing Awareness Exercise before
    and after other techniques, 95
  Ratio Breathing, 95
  reaction to news, 90–91
  team work, 110
  time spent on a technique, 94–95
  Triangles, 103–105
  "Wake Up!" (ANS Activation
    Technique), 102–103
  "We Need Energy!", 103–104
  "We Need to Relax!", 103–104
voice of unconscious-self, hearing, 39–44
  learning skill of interoception, 40–43
  relearning how to feel, 43–44
voluntary hyperventilation. *See*
  superventilation

W

"Wake Up!" (ANS Activation Technique),
  102–103
walking
  building your athletic CO_2 tolerance
    training program, 137
  CO_2-Focused Balanced Breathing,
    135–136
  Edge Breathing, 134
"We need energy!", 103–104
"We need to relax!", 103–104
whole self, 35

ABOUT THE AUTHOR

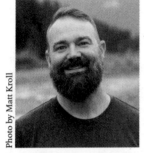

Photo by Matt Kroll

Jesse Coomer is one of the foremost voices in the world of breathwork today. In 2009 he began a life transformation mission that led him to discover how our physiology and psychology often conflict with the modern world and each other. In 2020, after studying with neuroscientists and breathworkers from various traditions, Coomer released his first book on breathwork, *A Practical Guide to Breathwork,* which offered the world a clear and concise understanding of how human physiology and breathing are interconnected. His book has sold thousands of copies all around the world and is one of the most recommended books on the topic of breathwork.

Today, Coomer is a human performance specialist, breathworker, and renowned speaker in the field of breathwork. He trains athletes, CEOs, first responders, military, and everyday people who seek to optimize their performance, reduce their anxiety levels, and live a healthier life.

>> READY TO TAKE THE NEXT STEPS? <<

Take the Language of Breath Online Course!

Enjoy an on-demand learning experience with Jesse as your guide and take your practice to the next level. The course includes guided breathing sessions and in-depth visual aids to ensure that you fully understand the Language of Breath Philosophy. This six-week course covers everything you will need to begin to form a powerful, positive relationship within yourself so that you can take actions to improve your life. Go to www.languageofbreathcollective.com for more information.

BECOME A CERTIFIED LANGUAGE OF BREATH BREATHWORKER
Train with Jesse Coomer, and learn to serve your clients using the complete Language of Breath system, providing more than just techniques. When you become certified, you become a member of the Language of Breath Collective, a community of Certified Language of Breath Breathworkers who collaborate and work together to bring breathwork to the world through safe and science-backed methods. For more information go to www.languageofbreathcollective.com or scan the QR code below.

ABOUT
NORTH ATLANTIC BOOKS

North Atlantic Books (NAB) is an independent, nonprofit publisher committed to a bold exploration of the relationships between mind, body, spirit, and nature. Founded in 1974, NAB aims to nurture a holistic view of the arts, sciences, humanities, and healing. To make a donation or to learn more about our books, authors, events, and newsletter, please visit www.northatlanticbooks.com.